The *Parents*™ Baby and Childcare Series combines the most up-to-date medical findings, the advice of doctors and child psychologists, and the actual day-to-day experiences of parents like you. Covering a wide variety of subjects, these books answer all your questions, step by important step, and provide the confidence of knowing you're doing the best for your child—with help from *Parents*™ Magazine.

"This is a book that expectant couples will first want to read from cover to cover, and then use as a handy reference throughout the months of pregnancy."

from the foreword by
David A. Kliot, M.D.

OTHER PARENTS™ CHILDCARE BOOKS
Published by Ballantine Books:

PARENTS™ BOOK OF BREASTFEEDING
PARENTS™ BOOK OF CHILDHOOD ALLERGIES
PARENTS™ BOOK OF TOILET TEACHING
PARENTS™ BOOK FOR YOUR BABY'S FIRST YEAR

Parents™ Book of Pregnancy and Birth

LEAH YARROW

BALLANTINE BOOKS • NEW YORK

Copyright © 1984 by Parents Magazine Enterprises, A Division of Gruner + Jahr, U.S.A., Inc.

All rights reserved under International and Pan-American Copyright Conventions. Published in the United States by Ballantine Books, a division of Random House, Inc., New York, and simultaneously in Canada by Random House of Canada Limited, Toronto.

Library of Congress Catalog Card Number: 84-90944

ISBN 0-345-30446-2

Manufactured in the United States of America

First Edition: December 1984

Illustrations by Linda Miyamoto

To my husband and my children, with love

Contents

Foreword		ix
Introduction		1
PART 1:	Maternity and Childbirth Care: Today's Options	3
PART 2:	Your Pregnant Body	54
PART 3:	Your Pregnant Self	115
PART 4:	Lifestyle	135
PART 5:	Preparing for Baby	161
PART 6:	Childbirth	202
PART 7:	The Postpartum Period	254
Afterword		278
Bibliography of Further Reading		281
Organizations for Expectant Parents		288
Index		291

Foreword

People often say to me, some with hardly concealed envy, "You really *do* enjoy being an obstetrician!" Basically it's true. Despite the unpredictable hours, the occasional sadness, and the conflicts inherent in any creative endeavor, the joy is contagious. People rarely reach the emotional heights they achieve when they give birth to a child. Pregnancy, too, is mostly a happy time—a dynamic period when a couple focuses sharply on their own vitality. Their motivation for learning is something most teachers would envy, for motivating students may be the hardest part of a teacher's job. Yet during pregnancy, motivation is "built in"—and there is so much to learn.

Today's consumer of obstetrical care is also demanding. We are in an age when couples are not only requesting choices, but are forced to make choices. And to make the ones that are right for them, they need solid information.

Parents™ *Book of Pregnancy and Birth* comprehensively covers the issues that are of interest to all expectant couples. Leah Yarrow has taken complex technical subjects and, without talking down to her readers, has made them easy to understand. She has presented the alternatives in obstetrical care so that the reader can make intelligent choices. She has dispelled the clouds of anxiety about what to expect during labor and delivery. She has charted the changes occurring in the fetus and the mother during each trimester. There is a discussion of the common discomforts of pregnancy and how to relieve them—handy information to have at the moment of need. And the discussion of preparing for the newborn—from purchasing clothing and equipment to choosing a feeding method—should be immensely helpful.

I am frequently asked by families under my care to recommend a book on pregnancy and birth. I usually suggest that they select a specific topic of interest, look it up in several books, then compare and evaluate the clarity of the explanations and choose the book they're most comfortable with. The clarity and completeness of *Parents® Book of Pregnancy and Birth* make it easy for me to recommend it. The information offered is well-founded, and the way it is presented is both fluent and reassuring. This is a book that expectant couples will first want to read from cover to cover, and then use as a handy reference throughout the months of pregnancy.

David A. Kliot, M.D.
Brooklyn, N.Y.

Introduction

When I became pregnant with my first child four and a half years ago, I knew little about pregnancy and birth. I didn't know anyone who was pregnant or who recently had a baby. I was both thrilled and scared, and I was eager for information. Like you, I turned to books for help in understanding what was happening to my body and to my emotions. I looked for authoritative information as well as personal insights into pregnancy, birth, and motherhood. To be honest, there wasn't a great deal out there. I learned about the physical changes of pregnancy and the mechanics of labor. I found a few firsthand accounts of birth and of the conflicting emotions of new parenthood. Two years later, when I was again pregnant, the reading material hadn't changed significantly, but having already had a baby, I needed it less.

You have chosen *Parents™ Book of Pregnancy and Birth* because you are seeking the same type of information and guidance that I sought. Generally, however, I felt that the books I read did not adequately prepare me for making choices about prenatal care or for the variations and subtleties of pregnancy, birth, and the postpartum period. Thus I set myself three tasks when I began work on this book: to be informative, to be honest, to be personal. *Parents™ Book of Pregnancy and Birth* addresses itself to the expectant mother and her spouse, but the information may be just as valuable to you even if you are not yet pregnant. In fact, if you are reading this book because you are considering having a baby, you will have even more time to weigh your options and to make thoughtful decisions.

I recall my two pregnancies as some of the happiest months of my life. They were filled with a delicious kind of expectancy, with admiration and newfound respect for *Mother* Nature, with new insights about myself, my family, and life, death, and creation. I felt caught up in the life-force in a profound way. *Parents™ Book of Pregnancy and Birth* reflects the depth of my feelings, together with the perceptions of other women who are pregnant or who have recently given birth. It is my intent not only to provide you with the latest professional advice and findings, but to unite you with other expectant and new mothers so that you can put your own experience into perspective. The content of this book is what I wish someone had said to me.

1. Maternity and Child Care: Today's Options

It often comes as a surprise that about the time you are celebrating the confirmation of your pregnancy, you must also be making some crucial decisions about the birth which is many months away. But when you've made the last phone call announcing the good news, it may suddenly hit you—you must decide who will provide your maternity care and where you will give birth. Both of these decisions involve a lot more than you may realize. Today, you have more options about how you will have your baby than ever before. Although they may seem a bit confusing at first, these options mean that you and your husband can find the caregiver and birth setting that suit you best.

Many women are so anxious to be under professional care that they often choose the caregiver first and only later give more thought to the type of birth setting they want. It's really very difficult to separate the two decisions. Almost always, the person who provides your prenatal care will be playing a considerable role in your labor and delivery. Your choice will probably determine where

3

the birth takes place and the manner in which it is conducted. So while you may feel pressured about finding a caregiver immediately, it really is important to make your selection carefully. Your choice, after all, is crucial to your health and satisfaction during pregnancy *and* birth.

Even before you consider who and where specifically, you must evaluate your own feelings and the options that are available. This isn't always easy, especially in a first pregnancy. "When I was pregnant with my first child, I read everything I could about pregnancy and birth, and I thought I was choosing wisely when I went to a recommended obstetrician affiliated with one of the best hospitals in the city," says one mother of two. "I wanted to be at that hospital because I wanted the best protection in case anything went wrong with me or the baby. I gave no real thought to anything other than safety, although I did ask if I would be able to nurse the baby on the delivery table. All the options I read about just didn't sink in. I didn't grasp the real differences between delivering in a delivery room and in a birthing room, between prepping and not prepping, rooming-in and not rooming-in. It's not that I wasn't thinking; I was. But it's difficult to evaluate choices and make decisions before you've had the experience of having a baby. Nothing went wrong with the birth, but now I tell expectant mothers how important it is to take your time choosing your caregiver and the place where you will deliver. Each detail does make a difference in how you feel about yourself and about the birth, and that affects how you feel about the baby, at least right at the beginning."

Another new mother says that she, too, was unprepared for making decisions about prenatal care and birth setting when she became pregnant. Like so many other newly expectant mothers, she asked a few friends for recommendations and chose one of the doctors because two of her friends recommended him. "It was afterwards, when I started going for checkups and had learned more about pregnancy and birth, that I realized that I probably would have chosen a different physician and hospital." The birth experience was not exactly what she and her husband had planned, because the doctor and hospital were more interventionist than they had thought or expected.

One of the most important reasons to carefully evaluate your feelings and the available options *before* selecting a caregiver and birth setting is to eliminate surprises during pregnancy and during labor. Too often we have trouble seeing ourselves as consumers purchasing a crucial service and blindly choose a caregiver without knowing his philosophy of pregnancy and birth. Your decision, of course, is not irreversible. Many women, for one reason or another, find that they want to change caregivers during pregnancy. But the more care you take in seeking a caregiver and birth setting that's right for you, the less likely it is that you'll have to switch in mid-pregnancy when continuity of care may be important to you. Surprises during labor are less easily rectified. You can't exactly change caregivers or locations when you're about to give birth. Because surprises can upset your equilibrium during labor, creating anxiety, it's best to know as much as possible beforehand.

To help you make an informed choice of caregiver and

birth setting, this section will discuss the many options that are available today. As you read, consider carefully what is important to you.

Family-Centered Maternity Care

The most exciting changes in the management of pregnancy and birth are reflected in what has come to be known as family-centered care. This is a philosophy that recognizes the emotional as well as the physical events of pregnancy and birth, and that seeks to strengthen and support the family as a whole. Parents are encouraged to take an active part in their health care, to become knowledgeable about the physical changes of pregnancy, to be responsible for good nutrition, and to play a decisive role in how they want their births to be managed. Family-centered caregivers are well versed in prepared birth techniques and attempt to manage labor and delivery with little or no medication and intervention. They recognize that parents need support and encouragement during labor and should be treated with respect and dignity. They are deeply aware of the importance of parent-infant bonding and exude an excitement about birth with warmth and compassion for the new parents.

The management of pregnancy and birth is in the midst of great change, and family-centered care is certainly the direction in which we are headed. Certain aspects of family-centered care are already well-established, especially father participation. Fathers are often welcomed to prenatal checkups and are especially encouraged to attend a visit to hear the baby's heartbeat. They attend prepared

Maternity and Childbirth Care: Today's Options

childbirth classes and learn how to coach and support their wives during labor. Nearly all hospitals have opened the labor and delivery rooms to fathers so that they can participate and share in birth. These changes are all fairly recent. Not too long ago, fathers were relegated to the role of accessory: accomplice in the act of creation, chauffeur to the hospital, and actor without a part, waiting in the wings during labor and delivery.

Family-centered care is popular because it is a dignified and pleasant way to have a baby. However, while we are moving in this direction, traditional practices are still common. Some caregivers still routinely view pregnancy and birth as medical problems to be managed. Women may not be as drugged and out of it during labor and delivery as they once were, but they may be treated like children, without respect, rather than like adults participating in a very natural and wonderful process. Some caregivers still leave husbands out of all aspects of prenatal care and separate them from their wives during labor and delivery. And there are still hospitals that treat only two parts of the family unit: mother and baby, and even they may be required to spend most of their time apart. In addition, there are caregivers and hospitals that pay only lip service to the concept of family-centered care, and it is important to be wary of them. Because family-centered care is popular, they feel they must at least appear to offer certain options to be competitive.

If you want a family-centered experience, you will have to seek it out. There *are* family-centered physicians and hospitals, as well as nurse-midwives and alternative birth centers which are inherently family-centered. The more you, the consumer, look for and demand them, the greater the changes in maternity care will be.

While family-centered care is first and foremost a philosophy, there are a number of specific options that are attributed to and that reinforce this personalized approach to childbearing. We will look at these now so you can better determine which ones may be right for you.

The Birthing Room

This is a combination labor and delivery room that is usually decorated to resemble a bedroom in a private home. A birthing room typically contains a single or double bed in which the mother labors and delivers, as well as a comfortable chair for the husband or support person. Some birthing rooms have bathrooms and also facilities for preparing or storing food. Because the birthing room is designed for couples anticipating an uncomplicated, prepared birth, there is usually minimal medical equipment. After delivery, parents and baby remain in the birthing room for some time, getting to know each other in a relaxed way.

Birthing rooms are being developed for two principal reasons. First, one of the chief complaints many women have about hospital deliveries is being transferred from the labor room to the delivery room when the baby's birth is imminent. Often the transfer is uncomfortable, coming during transition, which is the most intense and difficult phase of labor. The transfer can also be very awkward as the woman, between contractions, is assisted in getting her cumbersome and tired body onto the delivery table. Since a baby's arrival is not always as predictable as one would like, the transfer must sometimes be very speedy. This race down the hall to the delivery room can create anxiety in the mother, making it difficult for her to keep in control of contractions. At the very least, the transfer is annoying. In a birthing room, the mother is never moved from the bed she is laboring in unless an emergency arises, and she also has more freedom to assume the birth position she finds most comfortable.

Another reason for developing birthing rooms is to meet the demands of parents for a more personalized birth experience. Many couples object to the sterile atmosphere of the traditional maternity unit and feel that birth in the hospital often seems more a medical than a family event. As a result, some couples have turned away from hospital care. In fact, the perceived trend toward home birth during the last decade was instrumental in getting the birthing room concept going.

Certain criteria must usually be met in order to use a birthing room. Typically, you must be anticipating an uncomplicated labor and delivery, you must have attended prepared childbirth classes and plan to give birth with little or no medication, and you must not have any medical problem, such as high blood pressure or diabetes, that would put you at risk. In addition, if certain situations arise during labor, you may be moved out of the birthing room. For example, if you find that you need regional anesthesia, you probably would be transferred to a regular labor or delivery room.

The results of a childbirth poll published in the August 1982 issue of *Parents* magazine show that birthing rooms are very much underutilized. Of the more than 64,000 women who responded to the poll, only 5 percent delivered in a hospital birthing room. This figure would seem to indicate that many physicians are still reluctant to use the birthing room. In addition, there are hospitals that have such stringent requirements for women to be eligible for the birthing room that few actually can meet them. "I've seen hospitals that have 1,500 to 1,600 deliveries a year and only one or two patients a month in the birthing room," says Dr. Robert Block, a family-centered obstetrician from Turnersville, New Jersey.

The birthing room is not some far-out notion. The concept, in fact, has the endorsement of the five major professional organizations concerned with maternal and child health: the American College of Obstetricians and Gynecologists, as well as its Nurses Association, the American Academy of Pediatrics, the American College of Nurse-Midwives, and the American Nurses' Association. In 1978, these five organizations issued a joint statement on family-centered care in the hospital. They recommended a number of different options to personalize the hospital birth experience, including birthing rooms for an uncomplicated labor and delivery. The joint statement was subsequently endorsed by the American Hospital Association.

The fact that birthing rooms are underutilized is mentioned not to discourage you, but to encourage you to work a little harder to find a caregiver and birth setting that will support you. There are physicians and hospitals committed to family-centered care. At Manchester Memorial Hospital in Connecticut, for example, the majority of births are managed in the hospital's birthing rooms. It was at Manchester Memorial that the birthing room concept was first introduced in the U.S. in 1969. You should also know that most hospitals that do have birthing rooms only have one or two, and you may be out of luck if they're already occupied when you go into labor.

Bonding Time

One of the most fundamental aspects of family-centered care is having time to spend with your baby immediately after birth. In the past, when women were heavily sedated during labor, they were generally too groggy, if not unconscious, to hold and touch their babies until many hours after delivery. Today, however, with most women actively participating in birth, the opposite is true. Indeed, studies show that in a birth where there has been little or no medication, both mother and baby are ready to interact in a very meaningful way. And despite long hours of labor, most mothers find that they are too exhilarated to sleep and that they yearn to be with their babies. "After the baby was born, I felt sort of detached. It was hard to believe it was over and I was a mother. But then they handed her to me and I felt this tremendous emotional release," says one new mother. "I was entranced and I didn't want to let her go." The engrossment with her baby expressed by this mother is known as bonding, the tie that begins to bind parents and baby into a family unit.

Much of the key research on parent-infant bonding has been done by Drs. Marshall Klaus and John Kennell of Case Western Reserve School of Medicine in Cleveland. Klaus and Kennell have identified what they call a "sensitive period" for parent-infant contact during the first minutes and hours of life. They believe that during this time, the baby is in a "state of readiness" to begin forming a relationship with his parents. Research shows that a baby's senses are highly developed at birth and that he has unique capabilities to draw in his parents and enhance the attachment process. Klaus and Kennell note that a baby is usually in a state of quiet alertness for the first 45 to 60 minutes of life, after which he falls into a deep sleep for three or four hours. During this alert time, the baby is very responsive to his environment. He will turn his head if spoken to, lick the mother's nipple, and often begin suckling if offered the breast. In observing mothers and babies who were together during this "sensitive period," Klaus and Kennell noted that they interacted in particular ways. The mothers, for example, touched and stroked their babies, sought eye contact with them, and spoke to them in a special high-pitched voice. In turn, the babies made eye contact with their mothers and moved in rhythm to their voices, producing what some researchers have called a "synchronized dance" between mother and baby.

In follow-up studies, Klaus and Kennell compared mothers and babies who had early and extended contact with mothers and babies who didn't. According to their observations, the mothers in the first group breastfed for a longer period of time and were more affectionate, supportive, and attentive toward their babies at one month and one year. At two years, these mothers tended to talk to their children differently, asking more questions and giving fewer commands.

Some researchers object to the emphasis that Klaus and Kennell place on a "sensitive period" and its long-term significance. Despite the controversy over long-term effects, there is little dispute that early and extended contact should be encouraged and that it definitely has advantageous short-term effects. Being with your baby is probably the most pleasant way to spend the first hours after birth. Yet each meeting you have with your baby will forge your mutual relationship. The more you get to know one another, the more your attachment to each other will grow.

The research on bonding has had an impact on post-delivery routines. The most enlightened hospitals now make it possible for parents to spend at least 30 to 60 minutes in privacy with their baby after delivery. They allow skin-to-skin contact between mother and infant, and delay putting prophylactic drops into the baby's eyes until the parents have had an opportunity to hold and gaze at their newborn. These drops, which are required by law in most states, can blur the baby's vision and interfere with the eye-to-eye contact that many researchers believe is so important to parent-infant bonding.

The results of the *Parents* childbirth poll, however, indicate that many parents are still not being given the opportunity to spend much time with their babies after birth. Of the women who responded to the poll, 64 percent spent fewer than 30 minutes with their babies. One-third of the respondents spent fewer than ten minutes! But what's most telling is that 65 percent of the women said they would have preferred to remain with their babies longer than they were allowed. If spending time with your baby after birth is important to you and to your husband, keep this in mind when looking for a caregiver and birth setting.

Rooming-in

To further the attachment process, many hospitals today offer some type of rooming-in option. Those that are most progressive allow mother and baby to be together around the clock. Other hospitals offer a modified plan where the baby stays with her mother during the day, usually from early morning until late evening when the baby is returned to the nursery. Still others have a pared-down version of rooming-in that sets aside several hours each day when mother and baby are together continuously. The most enlightened hospitals also have unrestricted visiting privileges for fathers, which can be a decided advantage. A father, too, needs the opportunity to further his attachment to his baby.

Not so very long ago, mother, father, and baby were routinely separated during most of the hospital stay. The baby was kept in the central nursery, brought to her mother every four hours for a feeding, then returned to the nursery. The new father had even less contact with his baby, and because he was restricted to regular visiting hours, he didn't have a great deal of time with his wife either. This forced separation of mother and father often left each feeling isolated and lonely. And the separation of parents and baby frequently had another effect. When the new family arrived home, parents and baby were very much strangers to each other. A first-time mother had little idea of the baby's needs and often felt terribly insecure about taking care of her. In fact, some researchers believe that the separation of mother and baby during the hospital stay is a major factor in many cases of postpartum depression. There are, of course, still hospitals that routinely separate parents and baby, but their numbers are dwindling. The majority make it possible for the new family to spend time together during the hospital stay, although the amount of time can vary considerably.

With rooming-in and unrestricted visiting privileges for father, parents and baby have the opportunity to become acquainted with one another. Nurses are there to answer questions and to give support and assistance as the mother and father learn how to take care of their baby. By homecoming time, the parents have a better understanding of typical newborn behavior, as well as of their own baby's individual preferences and patterns. They feel more confident about basic baby-tending skills, such as diapering, bathing, and feeding.

Rooming-in is especially helpful if you plan to breastfeed. Because your baby is with you, you can easily feed her on demand, an important factor in getting nursing off to a good start. Breast milk is very easy to digest, and in the early weeks of nursing, a baby needs small, frequent feedings throughout the day. In addition, a mother needs these frequent feedings to establish her milk supply. If you have modified rooming-in, you will have to ask that the baby be brought to you for night feedings and that she not be given supplementary bottles when she's in the nursery. Despite their requests, however, some mothers find that their babies are given supplementary feedings. Then when the babies are brought to them, they are too full and sleepy to be interested in nursing.

Some mothers decide against rooming-in because they're afraid they'll get little rest and want to store up on it before going home to the 'round-the-clock demands of a newborn. Yet most women find that their babies spend much of the hospital stay sleeping (maybe even more than they'd like them to!) and that they're able to rest while the babies sleep. The rooming-in arrangement at many hospitals allows the mother to wheel the baby back to the nursery any time she feels tired or overwhelmed. Fifty-six percent of the women who responded to the *Parents* poll had some form of rooming-in, but an even greater number, 73 percent, said they would choose rooming-in if they had another baby.

Sibling Participation/Visitation

A fairly recent and mostly unstudied area of childbirth is the inclusion of children in the birth of their siblings. Most alternative birth centers offer this option, but at present, only a small proportion of hospitals do.

Advocates of sibling participation argue that childbirth is a normal and healthy part of life and that the joy of bringing a new family member into the world should be shared. They believe that if a child is included in the birth, he will feel closer to the baby and there will be less sibling rivalry. Others, however, feel that a child will interpret the events of birth differently from an adult. They fear that he may become overanxious about his mother's well-being and be more frightened than enthralled by the birth experience.

Sibling participation, of course, is a very individual matter. Not all parents would feel comfortable having their children present at birth. The hospitals and birth centers that offer this option emphasize that for it to be successful, both parents must want it, and the child must be carefully prepared. As part of the preparation, there is usually a tour of the birthing room and a film of a real birth. Special attention is given to preparing the child for the sights and sounds of labor and delivery, and for the fact that his mother will be unavailable to him. Virtually all birth centers and hospitals that allow sibling participation require that the child be accompanied by a support person who has sole responsibility for him. The support person is there to look after the child's physical needs, to answer his questions and anticipate any concerns he may have, and to go with the child to another room if he becomes restless or overly anxious.

Although a hospital may not allow children to be present at birth, it may offer some type of program to help prepare them for the mother's hospital stay. This usually includes a visit to the hospital, and there may also be a film or slide presentation of a birth. Practically all birth centers offer orientation programs for siblings, whether or not the parents plan to have them attend the birth.

While sibling participation in birth is controversial, there is little dispute that children should be allowed to visit their mothers and new siblings while they're in the hospital. For a young child, a mother's absence can be upsetting, no matter how well his parents may have prepared him. He may worry about her well-being and whether or not she is coming home. A mother, too, is often anxious about being away from her child. Letting him visit her is mutually beneficial, as it helps ease fears and concerns that each may have. Sibling visitation can also help a young child begin to adjust to the reality of a new baby, and it may help ease, although not eliminate, natural feelings of jealousy because the child has been made a part of this special family event.

Many hospitals today offer some type of sibling visitation option, although what's allowed can vary considerably. Some hospitals permit only one visit during the mother's stay; others allow one visit each day. Some set aside a special room where children and parents can be together; others permit children to visit in the mother's room. In some hospitals, children are allowed to have contact with the new baby; in others, they view the baby through the nursery window.

If you have a child, you may want to keep provisions for siblings high on your list of priorities when seeking a caregiver and birth setting.

Early Discharge

Until quite recently, mothers who had uncomplicated births routinely stayed in the hospital for three or four days. Although a three-day stay is still routine, there is more flexibility today about when a mother and baby can be discharged. The reason for this new attitude is due in part to the fact that so many women are preparing for birth and laboring and delivering with little or no medication. As a result, a prolonged hospital stay is not always necessary for recovery from birth, as it once was when women were heavily medicated. In addition, many new mothers are anxious to return to the comfortable, familiar surroundings of their own homes and to begin taking care of their babies by themselves.

Maternity and Childbirth Care: Today's Options

A growing number of hospitals are now offering an early discharge option. If the birth was uncomplicated and the mother and baby are in good health, both may leave the hospital as early as 12 or 24 hours after delivery. The new mother and baby may be visited at home by a nurse, usually on the first and third day following discharge. (Follow-up care is something that should be checked out ahead of time.) An added advantage to early discharge is that it helps reduce the hospital bill. Some insurance companies even offer a rebate as an incentive for choosing early discharge. At an alternative birth center, the parents and baby routinely leave the center within 12 to 24 hours after delivery. The center then provides follow-up care at home.

Some women consider staying in the hospital as long as possible to get some rest. This can be an advantage. Whether you are actually able to rest, though, depends on the particular hospital and even on your own personality. Hospitals can be disturbing. There's lots of hustle and bustle, with nurses and doctors coming in for routine examinations and tests; there is noise from the corridors and visiting hours several times a day. "I decided when I was pregnant that I was going to stay in the hospital the full three days so I could rest, be pampered, and get my head together before I went home with the baby. Boy, was I surprised by the hospital experience," says one new mother. "I didn't sleep at night because of the noise, the lights, and the feedings. During the day, there was always someone poking at me or the phone ringing. And my roommate had visitors even when I didn't."

Another advantage to staying in the hospital is learning from the nurses. If the hospital is well staffed, you will be able to get lots of baby care lessons from the nurses, and these can help make you feel more confident about going home. Many hospitals also offer baby care, bathing, and breastfeeding or bottle-feeding classes for new parents.

Leboyer Birth

Frederick Leboyer is a French obstetrician who has pioneered a method for easing the birth experience for the baby. Leboyer believes that the traditional way babies are brought into the world is unnecessarily traumatic. The harsh light and sounds of the delivery room, the feeling of open space, the abrupt handling—all are a shock for the baby, who for nine months knew only the close security of the warm, dark womb. To help make the transition gentler, Leboyer suggests that the birth environment be dimly lit and very quiet. As soon as the baby is born, he is placed on the mother's abdomen so that she can gently stroke and caress him. The umbilical cord is not cut until it stops pulsating; this way, the baby gets oxygen from both the cord and the lungs. After the cord is clamped and cut, the baby is given a warm-water bath, usually by the father. The bath recreates the aquatic environment of prenatal life and so provides another way to help ease the baby's transition from womb to world. All of this gentle handling results in a very calm and peaceful baby. Leboyer babies usually cry very little, if at all, during this immediate period of tender attention. Some have even been known to smile.

While Leboyer focuses his attention on the baby, the

ultimate aim is an optimal birth experience for everyone involved. When combined with a family-centered atmosphere, Leboyer's techniques can have a very positive influence on the attachment process. Many aspects of gentle birth are done routinely by family-centered caregivers. Leboyer's method, however, is still not universally accepted. Many caregivers object to the lowered lighting and see little merit in waiting to cut the umbilical cord. Perhaps the most objections are voiced over the Leboyer bath. Even some caregivers who practice the other aspects of gentle birth question whether the bath should be given. A newborn has some difficulty maintaining body temperature, and it is felt that the bath could result in the baby getting chilled. Those caregivers who are in favor of the bath say that this potential risk is easily overcome with proper attention to water temperature and by warmly wrapping the baby afterward.

If you are interested in learning more about Leboyer's philosophy, you may want to read his very eloquent book *Birth Without Violence* or Nancy Berezin's *The Gentle Birth Book*.

Physician/Hospital

While you may have more options today about how you will have your baby, most births take place in a hospital and are attended by a physician. This is due in part to the fact that nurse-midwives and alternative birth centers, while their numbers are increasing, are still relatively few and far between. In addition, many expectant parents are unaware of what choices are available; others feel most comfortable with the traditional way of having a baby—with an obstetrician for prenatal and childbirth care and a hospital for delivery. Ninety-eight percent of the women who responded to the *Parents* childbirth poll delivered in a hospital; 84 percent were attended by obstetricians and 10 percent by GPs and family physicians.

Because the family physician is a relatively new figure in medicine, you may not be as familiar with him as with an obstetrician/gynecologist. Nor is he to be confused with a general practitioner. Family practice is a specialty—it was certified by the American Board of Medical Specialties in 1969, and the first family physicians were certified in 1970. The family physician is trained in six disciplines: obstetrics and gynecology, pediatrics, surgery, internal medicine, psychology, and community medicine. He therefore can provide prenatal and childbirth care and also assume care of the new baby. And he can continue to provide care for the entire family. A growing number of young families are finding it advantageous to have one trusted physician provide most of their health care. Family practice has also become very popular among medical students; it is third after internal medicine and surgery as the preferred choice of specialty.

Team Versus Solo Practice

Physicians either practice alone or in groups, and there are advantages and disadvantages to each type of practice. A woman who chooses a doctor in solo practice feels most comfortable knowing that only one doctor will be providing her prenatal care and that he will be the one delivering the baby. The disadvantage to choosing a physician who practices alone is that there is no guarantee that he will always be available to answer questions. There is also no guarantee that he will be available to deliver the baby. He may be attending another birth at the time or he may be on vacation. Some doctors in solo practice will not plan a vacation within two weeks of the due date of any patient. If you are considering a physician who practices alone, you should ask what his policy is regarding this. In addition, finding a doctor in solo practice is more difficult than finding one in a group practice. The drawback to practicing alone is obvious—the physician is *always* on call.

Some women feel most comfortable with a physician in a group practice. While the doctor a woman chooses is her primary caregiver, there is someone on call 24 hours a day to answer questions and to handle emergencies. The disadvantage to group practice is that invariably you'll like one or two physicians more than the others. There is also no way of knowing who will be on call when you are ready to deliver. If your doctor has only one partner, there is more of a chance that your doctor will be attending your birth. The more partners your physician has, the smaller the chance that she will be delivering your baby. Even if they're not on call, some doctors in larger groups do try to deliver their own patients' babies. This is something you should inquire about if you are considering a physician in a group practice.

Of course, which type of practice a doctor has is not the most important criterion for choosing him, but it is helpful to understand the implications of each system. What's most important is that you have confidence in his abilities and that his philosophy of pregnancy and birth is compatible with your own. Another important consideration is his hospital affiliation; usually, a physician has privileges at one or two hospitals.

The Hospital

When we're looking for a physician, we often do not pay enough attention to the hospital with which she's affiliated. Yet where you give birth can have a substantial influence on the type of experience you have. This takes on added significance if you want a family-centered birth. Some expectant parents, in fact, choose a hospital first because it is family-centered, then look for a compatible doctor who has privileges at that hospital.

Most large medical centers are what are known as teaching hospitals. They are affiliated with medical schools, and their staffs include faculty members and students from those schools. A teaching hospital generally has the very latest technology and is the safest place to be if a mother or baby needs special care. However, because medical students are there to learn, a mother may be examined many times during her stay. Teaching hospitals may also be the slowest to change policy regarding family-centered care.

A small hospital has several advantages. Simply because of the smaller size and staff, it feels less impersonal. Policies, too, are often more flexible. A well-equipped small hospital can take care of routine problems, but transfer to a medical center may be required if a mother or baby develops serious complications.

Maternity and Childbirth Care: Today's Options

Most hospitals today offer some family-centered options, and some hospitals offer comprehensive family-centered programs. It's important to keep in mind, however, that family-centered care is first and foremost a philosophy. A hospital may have the most attractive birthing room in town, but it may very rarely be used. On the other hand, a hospital may not have a birthing room, but it may have a nursing staff that's experienced in prepared birth techniques, that supports and encourages parents during labor, and that is sensitive to their wishes. In the same vein, a physician may not have privileges at a hospital with a birthing room, yet he may embrace the wider meaning of family-centered care. He encourages parents to participate in the childbearing process and to help make decisions about their own health care. He doesn't routinely treat mothers as high risk, and he intervenes only when medically indicated.

Obstetrical Procedures

Not so very long ago, when a woman entered a hospital to give birth, she was routinely "prepped"—all the pubic hair was shaved, she was given an enema, and an intravenous drip was started. In recent years, however, the routine use of these and other procedures has been widely questioned, among mothers, childbirth educators, and health professionals alike. While such procedures are not as routine as they once were, they are still the norm in many hospital births.

These procedures have come to be thought of as hospital routines, but in reality, the hospital administration does not dictate that a woman be shaved or given an enema. The physician initiates these procedures either through his own standing orders or specific orders that he leaves regarding a particular case. Standing orders are instructions from the doctor to the hospital staff about how he wants his patients treated unless he issues orders to the contrary. For instance, a physician may include in his standing orders that all his patients admitted in labor be given an enema unless they are very close to delivering. Hospitals generally do not have specific rules about a woman having an IV or an enema. "Hospitals generally say that all patients must have a complete blood count and a urinalysis—that's it," says Dr. Robert Block, a family-centered obstetrician from Turnersville, New Jersey. "Almost everything is up to the doctor. The obstetrician takes precedence."

If a doctor refers to hospital policy, he may also mean policy as set by the group of obstetricians who are practicing at the hospital. This group sets policy about some major aspects of care. For instance, the group may decide that an obstetrician must be present when oxytocin is used to induce or to augment labor, or they will set criteria for who can do a cesarean delivery. "My experience is that not too much policy is set by the hospital administration," says Dr. Paula Hillard, assistant professor of obstetrics and gynecology at the University of Virginia School of Medicine. "Almost always, a lot of policy is a result of tradition. So if you try to get to the bottom of say, 'Who said every laboring woman needs an enema?' it's often a practice that's evolved for 20 years. It's seldom written as routine policy."

What this means is that there can be and should be

variation in the way different patients are treated. There are valid reasons for the use of these procedures in certain situations. Their use for every laboring woman is no longer considered necessary, especially by those professionals concerned with family-centered maternity care. If you wish to avoid these procedures, be sure to discuss the subject with any physician you may be considering.

Pubic Shave The original rationale for this was to provide a sterile environment for birth. It was assumed that pubic hair carried bacteria, which could lead to infection. However, studies have shown no difference in infection rates between women who are shaved and women who are not. In fact, some studies have shown that shaving can increase the chance of infection because of nicks and scratches in the skin. Women have always found the shave to be one of the more dehumanizing aspects of hospital births. There is also a lot of uncomfortable itchiness as the hair grows back. Still, 31 percent of the women who responded to the *Parents* poll had a complete shave; only 13 percent were not shaved at all. What has become most common is the so-called mini-prep. The hair between the vagina and the anus is either clipped with scissors or shaved. The rationale for this is that it makes it easier to do an episiotomy if one should be needed. An episiotomy is an incision made just prior to delivery to enlarge the vaginal opening. If you want to know more about this procedure, turn to page 242. Its routine use is also being questioned.

Enema The rationale for routine enemas is often twofold. First, by emptying the rectum and colon, there will be more space in the pelvic area. This, it is felt, can help augment labor, because the baby's head can press more effectively against the cervix, the opening of the uterus. It is also felt that if the rectum and colon are empty, the baby's passage through the vagina will be easier, although this theory has not been substantiated. The second common reason for giving an enema is so a woman will not hold back when it comes time to push the baby down and out of the birth canal. It is felt that a woman may not push as efficiently if she is worried about passing some fecal matter. This, however, is not necessarily so.

In some situations, an enema can be helpful. For example, an enema may help stimulate labor, and this could be useful if contractions are weak or very irregular. If a woman is already having efficient contractions, however, an enema can increase their intensity and frequency and make it more difficult for her to stay in control. Being given an enema when you are trying to cope with contractions can be extremely uncomfortable, and many women find it demeaning. In addition, nature often has its own solution. For many women, labor is preceded or accompanied by diarrhea, making an enema unnecessary.

A growing number of physicians are taking into account the needs and wishes of each laboring woman. Yet while the enema may not be as routine as it once was, it is still fairly common. Of the women who responded to the *Parents* poll, 55 percent had enemas.

IV Many physicians still expect all women to labor with an IV, although its routine use is debated. Doctors generally cite two reasons for using the IV. First, because a woman is often not allowed to eat or drink during labor, the IV is used to provide fluids and prevent dehydration. Second, the IV can be used to administer drugs should they be needed.

The rationale for prohibiting food and drink during labor is related to the use of anesthesia. If a woman is anesthetized or heavily sedated, there is the danger that she could aspirate undigested food. Aspiration is very serious and was a major concern when women were heavily sedated for labor and general anesthesia was used for delivery. Today, however, most women are preparing for birth and planning to labor and deliver with little or no medication. Because of this, a growing number of health professionals are urging a more flexible approach.

Certainly, if a woman is at risk or is planning to receive childbirth medications, an IV would be needed. If a woman is anticipating an uncomplicated, nonmedicated birth, however, starting an IV as soon as she is admitted to the hospital is unnecessary. An IV can always be started if needed—for example, if the labor should become unusually long or difficult. Some physicians allow mothers who plan to give birth with little or no medication to eat a light meal and to drink fluids while they're at home in early labor, and to have small amounts of broth or tea after they arrive at the hospital. A high-risk mother who may need a cesarean or a mother who anticipates taking childbirth medications should, of course, not eat once labor begins. But for a mother who is anticipating an uncomplicated, nonmedicated birth, a light meal in early labor is considered beneficial, as it will provide energy to help her get through labor without IV fluids. Most women find that once labor is well underway they are uninterested in food anyway. Many physicians and hospitals, however, still do not permit women to eat or drink once labor begins, although they usually allow ice chips to help ease parched lips and throats.

Many women find the IV inhibiting, both physically and psychologically. An intravenous stand is placed beside the labor bed and a needle is inserted into a vein in the mother's arm or hand. The stand has a bottle or bag containing sugar water, which runs through a tube and into the needle and vein. Because you are physically attached to the stand, your mobility is limited. In early labor especially, it's very beneficial to walk around, as this helps augment labor. As you get into active labor, you will probably feel more comfortable sitting or lying in bed. In addition, many women are afraid that if they make a wrong movement, the IV needle will become dislodged.

Of the women who responded to the *Parents* poll, 63 percent were given IV fluids. Looked at another way, 37 percent were not, which is an indication that policies regarding the routine use of IVs are beginning to change.

Electronic Fetal Monitoring (EFM) This is a relatively new procedure that has become increasingly routine in recent years. Electronic monitoring is used during labor to assess how the fetus is responding to uterine contractions and to detect signs of possible distress. It was originally developed for use with high-risk patients but has gradually been applied to low-risk patients too. It's been estimated that more than half of all labors are now monitored electronically. While physicians generally agree that electronic monitoring is a valuable diagnostic tool for patients who are at risk, there is disagreement over whether it should be used routinely for patients who are not at risk. Some doctors believe that all labors should be monitored to provide an extra margin of safety; others believe it should be used only when there are signs of risk to the baby or the mother.

Maternity and Childbirth Care: Today's Options

There are two basic types of electronic monitors: external and internal. With an external monitor, two belts are placed around the mother's abdomen, and on each belt there is a transducer. One transducer records the baby's heart rate and the other measures the frequency and duration of uterine contractions. With an internal monitor, the heart rate is recorded by an electrode that is attached to the baby's scalp, and the contractions are measured by means of a catheter that is placed in the uterus. With both types of monitors, the heart rate and contraction information is transmitted to a boxlike machine that provides a continuous and permanent record on a long strip of graph paper.

Of the two types, the internal monitor is more accurate and allows a mother more freedom of movement, but it is also more invasive. Before an internal monitor can be used, the cervix must be sufficiently dilated and the amniotic sac or bag of waters must be broken. If it hasn't ruptured spontaneously, it will be broken artificially. With internal monitoring, there is the risk of infection. The baby may also develop an abscess where the electrode was attached or the uterus may be perforated by the catheter, although these complications are rare. A mother's movement is more restricted with an external monitor and changes in position require readjustment of the transducers. An external monitor, however, can be used intermittently so that a mother can get up and walk about when not being monitored.

In labors that are not routinely monitored electronically, the baby's heart rate is checked at regular intervals with a fetoscope applied to the mother's abdomen. This is called auscultation. Those who favor routine electronic monitoring say that the drawbacks to auscultation are that it is not as accurate as EFM and that it provides information only at a certain point in time rather than continuously. Opponents of routine electronic monitoring argue that the information provided by the monitor may not always be an accurate indication of the baby's condition and may lead to unnecessary intervention, such as cesarean delivery. They note that since EFM was introduced, the cesarean rate has increased substantially. The reply to this is that the increase in cesareans is largely due to other changes in obstetrical practice and that as physicians become more familiar with EFM, they are able to interpret the information more accurately.

Expectant parents also have mixed opinions about electronic fetal monitoring. Some women find the monitor disturbing and complain that once it is attached, the focus of attention shifts from them and their bodies to the machine. Having a monitor is akin to having a television set in the room. All eyes are automatically drawn to it, and the needs of the laboring woman can be ignored unless she is fairly vocal. But some expectant parents find the monitor reassuring and helpful. Since the monitor can signal the beginning of a contraction before the woman is even aware of it, she can get a jump on the contraction by beginning her breathing and relaxation techniques. Husbands who watch the monitors more easily than they observe their wives can tell them that a contraction is beginning, letting them rest in between with the security that they won't be taken by surprise.

You should discuss electronic fetal monitoring with any physician you may be considering. Many of the doctors who believe in routine monitoring also recognize that

Maternity and Childbirth Care: Today's Options

EFM can influence the labor experience because it restricts a mother's position and movement, and they will use the monitor intermittently so that the mother can get up and walk about.

Making Your Choice

Finding a physician in whom you have confidence and whose philosophy of pregnancy and birth is compatible with yours can take a lot of work. It's easy to become overwhelmed and to settle for a doctor you're not sure you're happy with just to feel secure under someone's care. The matchmaking of a caregiver and an expectant couple is a delicate business, and the three of you will be married for almost a year. Your choice, remember, is crucial to your health and satisfaction during pregnancy and during birth. So know what it is you want and then seek it out. Whatever suits you best, there is a caregiver and birth setting out there to match.

If you have a gynecologist whom you see regularly and she also practices obstetrics, you may assume that she should be the one to provide your prenatal and childbirth care. This may be a very satisfactory arrangement—the physician knows you and your medical history, and you know and feel comfortable with her. Sometimes, however, pregnancy can change the type of personality we want in a caregiver. One young woman, pregnant with her first child, decided to switch from the OB/GYN she had been using for several years to a different OB/GYN for just that reason. "When I wasn't pregnant, I liked his acerbic manner and humor. I found it amusing and responded in kind," she explains. "But I realized after my first two prenatal visits that I wanted something different from a doctor whom I'd be seeing frequently and who'd be playing such a vital role in my pregnancy and birth. I wanted someone sensitive to me and how I was feeling, who wouldn't be quick with a retort but thoughtful in his response." This woman began investigating other possibilities and found a physician with whom she was very comfortable and satisfied. In addition, while you may know your OB/GYN's attitude about gynecological care, you may not know his philosophy of pregnancy and birth, and you will want to be sure that it is compatible with your own. You may be delighted to find that it is, or you may be surprised to find that it isn't and that you have to begin looking for a caregiver whose philosophy reflects what you want.

Friends and Relatives

The first people everyone asks for help in finding a physician are friends and relatives who have recently had babies. These are really the best sources of information about what individual doctors are like. Friends and relatives are usually willing to give details about how their pregnancies and births were managed: whether a particular physician was supportive or distant, patient or impatient, quick to use medical intervention or not. The more detailed your friends and relatives can be, the better you can assess the doctors they used. When you're getting their recommendations, however, it is essential to know

Maternity and Childbirth Care: Today's Options

what they wanted or expected from their physicians. The personality and philosophy of the person doing the recommending is as telling as the recommendation itself. Each expectant mother looks for different qualities in a caregiver, and what may have been a very satisfying experience for one woman may not be for another. The more you know about what the person wanted, the better you can evaluate her recommendation. Be sure to concentrate on specifics. If someone says, "Oh, use Dr. X. He was terrific," you should find out exactly why and how he was so wonderful. The same holds true for negative comments. If a friend or relative says, "Don't use my doctor," get her to tell you why. The reasons she didn't like him may very well be the reasons you would. Remember, too, to ask about a doctor's hospital affiliation—what family-centered options it offers and whether or not the staff is supportive. Also call the hospital yourself to get further information about particular policies and options. Hospitals with comprehensive family-centered programs welcome questions from expectant parents.

Organizations

Childbirth organizations and childbirth instructors are other excellent sources of information about physicians and hospitals and are usually quite knowledgeable about family-centered programs in a community. The International Childbirth Education Association, for example, is dedicated to family-centered care and has local chapters across the U.S. Such organizations, as well as childbirth instructors, are keenly aware of the importance of finding a compatible caregiver and birth setting, and you shouldn't hesitate to call upon them for assistance and advice. They come in contact with many physicians and hospitals and should also know whether or not other alternatives, such as nurse-midwifery care and alternative birth centers, are available in a community.

Parent support groups in your community are also good sources of information. For example, community YM-YWCAs and YM-YWHAs often have some type of parenting program, and the person who is in charge may be able to assist you. There are also private parent support groups, such as Family Focus in Evanston, Illinois, and the Mothers' Center in Westbury, New York. A childbirth organization or instructor, or a local Y, may be able to steer you to a private support group for additional information.

One final source of recommendations is a physician you know and respect. He may be able to recommend a caregiver and birth setting whose philosophy reflects what you are looking for.

Talking with friends and relatives and contacting organizations will not only give you a good idea of what family-centered options are available in your community, it will also help crystallize your own thoughts about the type of childbearing experience you would like to have. It may all sound like a lot of work—and to be honest, it isn't easy—but finding the caregiver and birth setting that suit you best will be well worth the initial effort.

Maternity and Childbirth Care: Today's Options

Preliminary Consultations

The recommendations of friends, relatives, and organizations, however, are not enough. You really must see for yourself whether you and a prospective physician share the same attitudes about pregnancy and birth and whether your personalities mesh. This can only be done through a preliminary consultation. Once you have the names of two or three doctors whose philosophy seems to indicate what you are looking for, make an appointment for you and your husband to visit each. Husbands today are so involved in pregnancy and birth that the physician's attitude toward your husband and his feelings toward the physician are important considerations. And consulting more than one doctor will give you the benefit of comparison and can help you feel more confident in the decision you finally make. One expectant mother who interviewed two physicians was originally reluctant, feeling silly and unsure of the real value of the two interviews, but she came away feeling that the meetings were tremendously productive. "There was a real difference between the two doctors," she says. "One was very supportive of my coming to talk and offered a great deal of information about himself without my having to ask the questions I'd prepared. I liked everything he said. The other told me my questions were 'obvious' and seemed irritated about the whole thing. On the basis of those interviews I knew exactly whom I would choose."

Before you can decide what to ask during the consultation, you must have given careful thought to exactly what you're looking for in a caregiver and to the type of birth experience you would like to have. The issues that most concern you will dictate many of your questions. All questions, if they are about something that is important to you, are legitimate to ask. In making your list, it's a good idea to categorize your questions so that the physician's responses give a total picture of his opinions on one subject. It is also a good idea to place high on your list the questions that are most important to you, since you may find that the questions are taking longer than you thought and the consultation must end before you're finished.

What to Ask Most physicians today are used to consultations, as more and more expectant parents are requesting them. The consultation is productive from the doctor's standpoint too. If there is going to be a personality conflict or a drastic difference in approach, it is best to know ahead of time. Just call the physician's office, explain that you are pregnant and considering this doctor for your care, and that you wish to make an appointment so that you can meet and talk with her before making your decision. The secretary's reaction may tell you something about the physician too. If she knows exactly what you're talking about and simply makes the requested appointment, you at least know the doctor is used to talking to expectant parents. If, however, she responds that the physician just doesn't have time to do that sort of thing, a consultation may be a waste of your time as well. You should also ask how much the doctor charges for a consultation and how much time she usually allows. If you know how much time you'll have, you can add or subtract questions from your list accordingly. Usually, a physician

Maternity and Childbirth Care: Today's Options 39

charges a set amount for a consultation. If you decide not to use her, you will be billed for that amount. If you do decide to use her, the amount will be included in the total sum she charges for prenatal and childbirth care.

Some doctors object to the way women approach them with questions during a consultation. They feel that some women are antagonostic and put them in a position where they must prove that they are good physicians or decent human beings. As with all relationships, you should be sensitive to the doctor, just as you expect and want her to be sensitive to you. If a physician-client relationship is not based on mutual respect and cooperation, it is counter-productive for both parties. A list of questions should not be a manifesto of demands. In the same vein, a doctor should be happy to answer any questions you may have. Besides, if you have done your homework by speaking with relatives, friends, and organizations, you should have a pretty good idea of the physician's approach to pregnancy and birth when you go for the consultation, as well as her hospital affiliation, what options it offers, and whether or not the physician utilizes and encourages those options.

The following are questions you may want to ask when interviewing a prospective physician. This list is not all-inclusive. However, if you want to be actively involved in your pregnancy and birth, the doctor's answers should give you a pretty good idea of whether or not you are both on the same wavelength.

1. What are your views about weight gain during pregnancy? Do you provide nutritional guidelines for your patients? (Weight gain should not be restricted during

pregnancy, and most experts recommend an average gain of between 24 and 28 pounds.)

2. How do you feel about prepared childbirth? How do your prepared patients usually fare during labor? (If you plan on a drug-free birth and he says most mothers usually end up requesting medication, this may not be the physician for you.) Do you recommend any particular method of prepared childbirth? Do you have an instructor associated with your practice, or do you recommend childbirth instructors?
3. How do you feel about fathers attending prenatal visits?
4. What are your standing orders regarding pubic shaves, enemas, IVs, and electronic fetal monitoring? Do you take into account the individual needs and requests of each laboring woman? (If he doesn't, he may not be right for you.)
5. When do you arrive at the hospital after a mother in labor has been admitted? What is your role during labor? How much can I expect to see you? (Most physicians do not spend very much time with their patients during labor, but many women wish that they did. Asked what their doctors could have done better, 36 percent of those who responded to the *Parents* poll replied, "Spent more time with me.")
6. In the event that childbirth medications become necessary, what do you use? What are the effects of these medications? What are the risks?
7. What do you consider indications for an episiotomy? Do you do episiotomies routinely?
8. What may be indications for a cesarean delivery? If a cesarean becomes necessary, can I be given regional

anesthesia so that I can be awake for the birth? Will my husband be able to remain with me during the cesarean?

9. What hospital are you affiliated with? What family-centered options does the hospital offer—birthing rooms, bonding time, rooming-in, unrestricted visiting privileges for fathers, sibling visitation, early discharge, Leboyer birth? How do you feel about these options? Do you encourage their use? If the hospital has a birthing room, do you use it? How long will my husband and I be able to remain with our baby after birth? If I find that I would like to leave the hospital early, are you in favor of this? Does the hospital provide tours of the maternity facilities? How soon can my husband and I take such a tour?

10. If the doctor is in solo practice: Who covers for you when you're not available? What are the chances that you will be delivering my baby? If he is in a group practice: Will I meet all the physicians? What are the chances that you will be delivering my baby?

11. What are your office hours? Do you have a call-in hour for nonemergency questions? How can you be reached if an emergency arises during nonoffice hours?

12. What is your fee for prenatal care and vaginal delivery? What is your fee for cesarean delivery?

Before arriving at the preliminary consultation, you've done a lot of work determining what kind of care is important to you. From the consultation, you'll be able to assess the doctor's overall attitudes, as well as specific responses to your questions. You'll have to consider how well you liked her in general and whether there seemed to be some flexibility in her approach. You don't have to agree 100 percent with a physician for her to be the right one for you.

The Nurse-Midwife

The nurse-midwife is becoming a popular choice for prenatal and childbirth care. A certified nurse-midwife is a registered nurse who has completed a postgraduate program in obstetrics and who has passed a national certification exam developed and administered by the American College of Nurse-Midwives. The nurse-midwife is trained to manage normal pregnancies and births and to do routine gynecological care, including family planning.

As important as the nurse-midwife's medical expertise is her philosophy of pregnancy and birth. She encourages parents to help make decisions about their own health care, and she tries to accommodate their wishes within the guidelines of safety. She emphasizes preventive care through good nutrition and adequate rest and exercise, and she offers assistance and advice on breastfeeding and infant care. She discusses the emotional adjustments of pregnancy and new parenthood, and she is keenly responsive to the emotional needs of the laboring woman. She is trained in prepared birth techniques and in helping women give birth with little or no medication or medical intervention. It is this personalized, family-centered approach to childbearing that is making nurse-midwifery care so attractive to a growing number of expectant parents.

"I felt very supported by the midwives and was comfortable about asking questions I may not have asked a doctor," says one mother who used an in-hospital nurse-midwifery program. "It was very important to me that the midwife be with me throughout labor and delivery, that I would have her support. The midwives were all women, and that made a difference too. Many had children and had gone through the experience. They gave extra support and understanding." Many expectant mothers who use nurse-midwifery care say they appreciate the woman-to-woman relationship and feel at ease asking questions. Perhaps the most frequently cited advantage, though, is that the nurse-midwife remains with the mother and father during labor.

Nurse-midwives practice in a team relationship with a physician, although they often have a good deal of autonomy. Physician backup is necessary for consultation or referral in case a complication arises. Many nurse-midwives work in the maternity clinics of large medical centers; others staff in-hospital midwifery programs for private patients, such as the one at Roosevelt Hospital in New York City. There, a team of nurse-midwives works quite autonomously within the maternity unit, providing prenatal and childbirth care to their patients in a family-centered environment. Staff physicians provide obstetrical backup. Roosevelt was the first voluntary hospital to offer a private midwifery program, which began in 1974. Another pioneering hospital in the utilization of nurse-midwives is Booth Maternity Center in Philadelphia. Booth is a free-standing maternity hospital where nurse-midwives and physicians work as a team providing inclusive family-centered care.

In addition to midwifery programs within a hospital

setting, many nurse-midwives staff alternative birth centers, an option we will look at in a moment. And a growing number of physicians are finding it advantageous to bring nurse-midwives into their private practices to help provide care for low-risk patients. The physicians then have more time to devote to high-risk mothers, who need their specialized skill and training. The midwife's role in private practice depends largely on the doctor with whom she's associated, as well as on the policy of the hospital where he has privileges. In some situations, the nurse-midwife provides prenatal care only; in other situations, she provides prenatal care and also attends deliveries.

The first American school of nurse-midwifery was started in 1931 by Maternity Center Association, a voluntary health agency in New York City. The school was eventually transferred to Downstate Medical Center–Kings County Hospital in Brooklyn, New York, to become the first nurse-midwifery program in a major hospital with a university affiliation. Because of restrictive laws, however, there were few opportunities for American nurse-midwives to utilize their skills and training. Many turned to teaching or to public health; some went to other countries where trained midwives have traditionally played an important part in the management of pregnancy and birth. The World Health Organization estimates that 80 percent of the world's babies are delivered by midwives. While midwives play an essential role in developing countries, they are also an integral part of the health-care systems of more technologically advanced nations. In Holland, France, England, Norway, Denmark, Sweden, and Israel, for example, midwives are respected members of the obstetrical team.

Maternity and Childbirth Care: Today's Options 45

It wasn't until the 1960s that the organized medical system in the U.S. began to open its doors to the nurse-midwife. Even then, it was a very tiny opening. Demographers were predicting a baby boom as all the babies born after World War II started to come of age. Would there be enough physicians to meet this coming demand? Many health professionals thought not, and a few began calling for more nurse-midwifery programs and a greater utilization of nurse-midwives in hospital clinics. American nurse-midwives, however, would have to wait until the 1970s before they would gain wider acceptance. A major reason for this increased recognition was a joint statement issued in 1971 by the American College of Obstetricians and Gynecologists, its Nurses Association, and the American College of Nurse-Midwives. According to the statement, nurse-midwives, working as part of a healthcare team and under qualified medical direction, "may assume responsibility for the complete care and management of uncomplicated maternity patients." Many believe that this team approach is the best way to assure that all women receive high-quality maternity care. With the nurse-midwife managing normal pregnancies and births, the obstetrician has more time to devote to high-risk mothers.

As of early 1984, there were approximately 3,000 certified nurse-midwives in the U.S., as well as 28 nurse-midwifery educational programs with about 250 new graduates each year. Most of these programs, which range from one to two years, are university-affiliated. The United States Air Force has its own nurse-midwifery program at Andrews Air Force Base in Maryland.

When nurse-midwives were originally accepted into the U.S. medical system, it was mostly to provide maternity care for clinic patients. What has happened, however, is that nurse-midwifery care has become an attractive alternative for private patients who are seeking the type of family-centered care nurse-midwives are trained to give. If you would like to know if nurse-midwifery care is available in your area, you can write to the American College of Nurse-Midwives, 1522 K Street, N.W., Suite 1120, Washington, D.C. 20005. Childbirth organizations and instructors should also be able to help you.

The Alternative Birth Center

A growing number of expectant parents seeking a family-centered experience are finding the alternative birth center (ABC) the answer to their needs. The birth center is a relatively new concept. The fact that it is a recent development may help explain some of the confusion about just what a birth center is or should be. The term has been used to describe a variety of services that are actually quite different from one another. It is frequently applied not only to out-of-hospital centers but to alternative birthing facilities within a hospital—these may range from a simple birthing room to a comprehensive family-centered program that may or may not include prenatal care. As used here, however, the term birth center is based on the original concept—a free-standing facility, outside a hospital setting, that offers complete prenatal and childbirth care to low-risk mothers who are planning a prepared birth with little or no medication. Many expectant parents who choose to use an ABC do so because they want to take an active part in their own health care and because they want to give birth in a homelike environment, outside an institution, where the emphasis is on as little intervention as possible. A birth center is usually less expensive than conventional physician/hospital care and may even offer more in terms of classes and follow-up.

Many alternative birth centers are staffed by nurse-midwives, with physician and hospital backup in case complications arise; others are staffed by physicians. Birth centers usually offer a comprehensive parent education program, which covers not only preparation for birth but also many facets of pregnancy and new parenthood, as well as breastfeeding and infant care. The emphasis on education is essential to the birth center concept. Parents are considered members of the health-care team and are encouraged to take part in the decision-making. Also essential is the recognition that childbearing is a family affair—and family means more than the expectant mother and father. Children are welcomed to prenatal visits and most centers allow them to be present at birth, along with other relatives and close friends. The staff tries to accommodate parents' wishes about the type of birth experience they would like to have, within, of course, the guidelines of safety. Parents and baby are not separated after birth; they stay together until they leave the center, often within 12 hours after delivery. The center then provides follow-up care during the first week at home.

Because alternative birth centers only provide care for low-risk mothers, women are carefully screened for medical complications, from the first prenatal visit and throughout pregnancy and labor. If a complication either is expected because of a mother's medical history or is evident upon the first examination, she will not be accepted into the program. If a problem arises during pregnancy, she will be referred to a physician, and if it occurs during labor, she will be transferred to a hospital. All birth centers should have access to obstetrical consultation and a backup hospital.

The first free-standing birth center was opened in 1975 in New York City. Called the Childbearing Center (CbC), it is operated by Maternity Center Association, the voluntary health agency that started the first American school of nurse-midwifery in 1931. The Childbearing Center is staffed by nurse-midwives and three obstetricians who are in private practice serve as consultants. A mother is examined by one of the physicians at the beginning and end of pregnancy, and he can be called upon if a problem arises. The nurse-midwives provide all prenatal care and attend all births. In addition, they encourage expectant parents to take an active part in their own health care. Before each appointment, for example, a mother weighs herself, tests her own urine, and enters the results on her chart. The CbC program includes touch relaxation and prepared childbirth classes, as well as classes for siblings. A room with toys is provided to entertain children when they accompany their parents on prenatal visits. The labor and delivery setting is designed for the parents' comfort and to encourage mobility. There is a lounge with couch, rocking chair, TV, and kitchen facilities; a patio which can be used during warm weather; and two homelike birthing rooms. There are no routine procedures such as IVs, enemas, and pubic shaves, and a mother is free to assume the birth position she finds most comfortable. Should a problem arise during labor, the CbC's backup

Maternity and Childbirth Care: Today's Options 49

hospital is 11 minutes away by ambulance. A pediatrician examines the baby before she leaves with her parents and a public health nurse visits the new family during the first five days at home. The family returns to the center about a week after delivery and then again for the six-week postpartum checkup.

Because of the careful screening techniques, 85 percent of the women who labor at the Childbearing Center deliver there, according to Ruth Watson Lubic, a nurse-midwife and general director of Maternity Center Association. About 20 percent of the families who begin prenatal care at the CbC transfer out before labor begins; either they become ineligible for medical reasons or they withdraw for personal reasons.

Dr. Lubic, who has been a motivating force behind the birth center concept, has described birth centers as "maxi-homes" and not "mini-hospitals"—and in fact, many centers are located in what were once private residences. Put another way, a birth center is not a slimmed-down hospital but a homelike setting that has been expanded to include basic life-support equipment for a mother or infant requiring transfer to a hospital. Centers do not have the full range of technology found in the modern hospital: electronic fetal monitors, ultrasound devices, cesarean section capability, intensive care units, and a wide array of anesthetics and analgesics. The absence of this technology has prompted criticism by some medical professionals and organizations, although the criticism has receded somewhat after several years of successful birth center operation. The failure to provide this technology, say some physicians, creates a needless risk for a mother and baby. The response of those who support the birth center concept is that if intervention of this kind is really necessary, mother or baby should be—and will be—transferred to a hospital.

By early 1984, there were an estimated 125 to 150 alternative birth centers already open or in the planning stage. None of them are affiliated with Maternity Center Association, but its Childbearing Center often serves as a model and the agency frequently provides start-up advice and assistance in planning. Although we might tend to think of birth centers as being an option only in trendier, large metropolitan areas, they can be found in suburban and rural areas as well.

If you find the birth center concept of interest, perhaps the best way to decide whether or not it's right for you is to visit a center. Most birth centers have regularly scheduled orientations, which include a tour of the facilities and ample time to ask questions. Childbirth organizations and instructors should know whether there is a center in your area. Or you can write to the National Association of Childbearing Centers. This is an office set up privately in 1981 to pool information from birth centers and make it available to the public. Its address is Box 1, Route 1, Perkiomenville, Pennsylvania 18074.

Home Birth

The home birth movement began in the early 1970s as the response of some couples to what they viewed as the highly interventionist obstetrics practiced at the time. Those who sought a home birth wanted to avoid such routine hospital procedures as pubic shaves, enemas, IVs, drugs, stirrups for delivery, separation of mother and father, and separation of mother and baby. They wanted to give birth in familiar surroundings with the support of family and friends. While the home birth and alternative birth center movements have had their impact on hospital births, making many more flexible and family-oriented, the popularity of home birth has grown slowly but steadily. Today, between 30,000 and 40,000 babies are born at home each year.

In choosing a birth setting, safety is one of the principal issues for every expectant parent. Opponents of home birth maintain that it is unsafe. The American College of Obstetricians and Gynecologists, in its statement on home birth, says: "Labor and delivery, while a physiologic process, clearly present potential hazards to both mother and fetus before and after birth. These hazards require standards of safety which are provided in the hospital setting and which cannot be matched in the home situation."

Proponents of home birth, however, dispute the safety issue. They maintain that hospitals are not the safest place to have a baby. Routine interventions can have a profound and potentially detrimental effect on labor and delivery. Most babies in the United States are delivered in hospitals, yet it is ranked 19th in infant mortality in the world, according to recent statistics compiled by the World Health Organization. Many of the countries with lower infant mortality rates than the U.S. have comprehensive home obstetrical services. "Home birth is not what it was 30 years ago," explains Dr. Mayer Eisenstein, medical director of Family Practice Unlimited, a comprehensive health service in Chicago that offers professionally attended home birth. "You're not taking your life into your own hands anymore. Technology has enabled us to bring sophisticated equipment—plasma expanders, portable oxygen, resuscitation equipment, etc.—into the home. Don't forget," he adds "you can't perform surgery in ten minutes in the hospital. You have to assemble the operating team, call the anesthesiologist. This can take a lot of time."

Fear of the hospital setting itself can also be enough to complicate a woman's labor. Dr. Eisenstein, who is a founding member of the American College of Home Obstetrics, calls it the "home court advantage." In sports, he explains, the team playing at home is considered to have an advantage. So, too, does the woman who labors and delivers at home.

But even its most avid supporters acknowledge that not every woman can give birth at home, even if she wants to. Although the majority of pregnancies are normal, complications can arise that may necessitate a hospital delivery. The physicians at Family Practice Unlimited, like the staff at the Childbearing Center, carefully screen their patients. They are skilled at recognizing any sign of a problem before an emergency. Because of this extensive screening, few women need to be transferred from home to hospital during labor.

If you are considering home birth, you should seek the best care available. Finding a physician or nurse-midwife to attend a home birth is not easy. You need a caregiver who can offer expert prenatal care and screening, who has hospital backup (and, in the case of a midwife, physician backup) in case of complications, and who is knowledgeable about newborn care. For more information about home birth and for assistance in finding a physician, con-

Maternity and Childbirth Care: Today's Options

tact the American College of Home Obstetrics, P.O. Box 25, River Forest, Illinois 60305.

Postscript

Your final choice of caregiver and birth setting will to a great extent be based on feelings, but if you've really investigated your options, you can have confidence in your instincts. You will have read, thought, discussed, and arrived at a decision that is right for you. Your choice may not be what you thought it would be when you first began thinking about prenatal and childbirth care—which only proves how much time and effort you'll have given to making that choice. You and your husband can be proud of yourselves for giving each other and your unborn baby the best possible gift of all—good prenatal care with a caregiver who is best suited to your personalities, needs, and wishes, and a birth setting that will make you feel the most comfortable and relaxed.

2. Your Pregnant Body

At probably no other time in your life will your body undergo so many different changes in such a relatively short period of time as it will during pregnancy. The main purpose of these changes is to nourish and protect your baby, and the changes that he will experience are even more phenomenal. By the end of this nine-month period, he will weigh five or six billion times more than when he began life as a single cell, and that one cell will have multiplied into 200 million cells.

Your task during these nine months is twofold: to look after your baby's health and to look after your own. There are many things that you can do to help promote your baby's health. Eating right and gaining adequate weight are two that are very important. Many studies have shown that a well-balanced diet and sufficient weight gain during pregnancy have a direct relationship to the baby's proper growth and development. Equally essential is being aware of the potential risks that drugs, cigarettes, and alcohol pose to the baby and to act accordingly. At one time, it was thought that the placenta served as a barrier, filtering out most harmful substances before they reached the baby. Now we know that any substance—good or bad—can cross the placenta and enter the baby's bloodstream. Getting regular prenatal care is one more important precaution that you can take. The vast majority of pregnancies are normal and medically uneventful. There is, however, a slight possibility that a problem could arise, and this is why you need regular care throughout pregnancy. Thanks to medical advances, many complications can be detected early and successfully managed.

This section will take a closer look at the bodily changes that pregnancy brings and at the amazing growth and development of the unborn baby. And it will focus on what you can do to help promote your health and your baby's. This is a job that most women take on with eagerness and dedication. There are, after all, few jobs in life that are as personally rewarding as having a child.

Body Changes

By the time you miss your first menstrual period, monumental changes are already taking place. You won't look different, but you may feel different. You may find yourself nodding off at eight P.M. when you normally don't go to bed until 11, or you may feel just a bit nauseous when you get up in the morning. The fatigue or queasiness may add to your suspicion that something is up.

Fortunately, bodily changes don't happen all at once but take place gradually over the nine months of pregnancy. Actually, a pregnancy lasts about 266 days from the time of conception, or 280 days from the first day of the last menstrual period. This is how a due date is usually calculated, since it is difficult to know on exactly what day a woman conceived. A simple way to estimate your due date is to count back three months from the first day of your last period and then add seven days. A due date, of course, is only an estimation. Even if you knew the day on which conception took place, your baby might be born before or after the 266thday. Few babies arrive ex-

---

Your Baby's Development

The First Trimester

By one week after conception, your baby has already developed from a single cell into a cluster of more than 100 cells. This cluster of cells is called a blastocyst and is about the size of the head of a straight pin. On about the ninth or tenth day, the blastocyst firmly embeds itself into the lining of the uterus. By the time implantation takes place, the cells number several hundred, and they have already begun to differentiate. The inner cells will develop into the embryo and the outer cells will develop into the placenta, umbilical cord, and amniotic sac. The placenta will carry oxygen and nutrients to the baby through the umbilical cord and carry away the baby's waste products. The amniotic sac and fluid will serve as a shock absorber, helping to cushion the baby against jolts and pressures.

Embryonic development proceeds rapidly. By the end of the first month, a primitive heart has formed and already begun to beat. The brain has started to develop, and the head has markings where facial features will soon appear. There is a rudimentary digestive tract and also primitive kidneys and liver. At month's end, the embryo is about ¼ inch long and looks very much like a tiny seahorse with the relatively large head almost touching the "tail." The tail is actually an

Your Pregnant Body

extension of the spinal column and will gradually disintegrate and disappear.

During the second month, the embryo begins to take on a more human form. Limb buds grow into arms and legs; then the hands and fingers, feet and toes begin to form. By month's end, finger and footprints are already engraved. Ears, eyes, nostrils, and lips become clearly visible. The tongue forms and buds for the primary teeth appear in the gums. Brain development continues at a rapid pace. By the end of the month, the embryo is about 1¼ inches long and weighs about 1/30 of an ounce. Almost all of the internal organs and systems have developed, although they are still primitive and need further refinement to be completely functional. The end of the second month marks the end of the embryonic period. Your baby is now a fetus.

During the third month, bone begins to form and the baby becomes very active. By month's end, she can kick, make a fist, curl her toes, and turn her head, although you will be unaware of her movements. The eyes, which were far apart on the head, move closer together, and the nose and outer ear completely form. Eyelids, however, are fused and will not open until the sixth month. The baby can pucker her lips, open and close her mouth, even swallow. Fingers and toes are well formed, and soft nails begin to grow. The external genitals form, and the baby's sex can be determined. Internal reproductive organs are also developing. By month's end, the baby weighs about 1 ounce and is about 3 inches long. He is basically complete and looks very much like a miniature human being.

The Second Trimester

While the first three months of life are a period of rapid development, the second three are a time of rapid growth. During the fourth month, your baby will experience a growth spurt that will not be duplicated during any other month of prenatal life. By month's end, she may have doubled her length and increased her weight sixfold. The baby's heart is now pumping about 25 quarts of blood through her body each day, and her heartbeat will soon be strong enough to detect with a fetoscope. The baby's posture is becoming more erect and her head is more in proportion to her body. She is becoming increasingly active, rolling and turning in the bag of waters.

By the beginning of the fifth month, your baby may have a new activity: sucking her thumb. She will have sleep and wake patterns that are similar to a newborn, and she may respond to an outside noise, such as loud music or a banged door. Her body may be covered with a fine down, which is called lanugo, and hair will begin to grow on her head and brows. Her eyelids may also be fringed with lashes. By month's end, she may weigh almost 1 pound and be almost 12 inches long.

During the sixth month, the baby's eyelids open to reveal well-formed eyes, and the baby can move her eyes up and down and from side to side. Her skin is red and wrinkled, with little fat beneath it, but it is protected with a whitish, creamy substance called vernix caseosa. The buds for the permanent teeth are beginning to form high up in the gums, and there is an abundance of taste buds inside the baby's mouth and on her tongue. By the end of this month, the baby's posture is quite erect, and she may be about 2 inches longer and about 1 pound heavier. Her brain is entering a critical period of growth, which will continue throughout the rest of prenatal life. If the baby were born at this time, she would be able to make a crying sound.

The Third Trimester

Growth begins to slow down during the last three months but the baby's systems continue to mature for independent life. At about seven months or 28 weeks, the baby is considered viable, which means that her systems are sufficiently developed and she has a good chance of surviving if born prematurely. She will, however, need intensive medical care and

Your Pregnant Body

the controlled environment of an incubator. One of the main problems is the immaturity of the lungs. At seven months, too, there is little fat beneath the skin, and the baby will have difficulty maintaining body temperature.

During the eighth and ninth months, the lungs continue to mature, and fat deposits form beneath the skin. The baby will gain about ½ pound a week during this period, and the fat deposits will smooth out the wrinkled skin. At birth the average baby weighs 7½ pounds and is 20 inches long.

With each passing month, space in the uterus becomes increasingly cramped, and the baby's kicks and pokes become more vigorous and visible. Most babies settle into a head-down position during the seventh or eighth month. In a first pregnancy, the baby often "drops" or becomes engaged at about the 36th week. This means that the head or presenting part has descended into the pelvis. In a few more weeks, the baby will make her entry into the world.

actly on schedule. Most make their entry within two weeks before or after their expected dates of arrival.

Expectant mothers are usually eager to know what bodily changes might be expected as pregnancy progresses. And they're often just as curious about how their babies are growing and developing. The following timetable gives an overview of fetal development and of maternal body changes for each of the trimesters.

Your Changing Body

The First Trimester

Many of the bodily changes that occur during pregnancy are controlled by two hormones—estrogen and progesterone. For example, one of the first changes that you may notice is a fullness and tenderness of the breasts, and this is largely the result of the action of these hormones. Very early in pregnancy, they alert the milk-making structures to begin developing in preparation for breastfeeding. The principal function of estrogen and progesterone is to help maintain the pregnancy. Estrogen, for example, stimulates the development of uterine blood vessels, and one of the functions of progesterone is to help keep the uterus from contracting too strongly. Both of these hormones will be produced by the placenta throughout pregnancy.

While they help to maintain the pregnancy, estrogen and progesterone can also contribute to certain discomforts, particularly during the early months when the body is adjusting to their rapid increase. Increased hormonal levels, for example, cause the smooth muscles to relax, and this can contribute to constipation and the frequent need to urinate which are common complaints in early pregnancy. Increased hormonal levels also cause a relaxation of pelvic ligaments, and this can lead to lower backache. Nausea is another common

Your Pregnant Body

discomfort that may be due largely to hormones—particularly the hormone HCG. Levels of this hormone are very high during the first trimester, which, coincidentally, is the time when most women are bothered by nausea. When levels of HCG begin to taper off, nausea usually subsides. (HCG, by the way, forms the basis of most pregnancy tests.) What about the fatigue that is so common in early pregnancy? It, too, can be mostly attributed to increased hormonal levels, particularly progesterone.

While many changes are taking place within the uterus and it is expanding, this growth will not be outwardly noticeable until you get into the second trimester. During the early months, the uterus is confined to the pelvis. By two months, the fundus, or top of the uterus, may be about a quarter of the way to the navel; by three months, it may be halfway to the navel.

You may, however, notice other outward signs of pregnancy. As the milk-making structures develop, for example, and the breasts enlarge, the skin begins to stretch and you may see a fine network of veins beneath it. During this trimester, too, the nipples and areolae may begin to enlarge and get deeper in color. This increased pigmentation is thought to be due to increased hormonal levels. You may also notice tiny nodules on the areolae. These are the glands of Montgomery. They secrete a solution that lubricates and protects the nipples during nursing. One more thing that may be noticed during this trimester is an increase in vaginal discharge.

The Second Trimester

As you enter the middle months of pregnancy, the discomforts of the first trimester usually subside or disappear. Hormonal levels stabilize, the pregnancy becomes an established condition, and you will have adjusted to it physically. Most women find the second trimester to be the most pleasant and often feel a new surge of energy and well-being.

During this trimester, the uterus will begin to enlarge at a regular rate, and it will become too big to remain entirely within the pelvis. By four months, the fundus, or top of the uterus, may be three-quarters of the way to the navel; by five months, it may be at the navel. As the uterus enlarges, the pregnancy will begin to show, and this usually happens during the fourth or fifth month. At about four and a half months, you may feel the baby's movements for the first time. The perception of fetal movement is called quickening, and the first movements may feel very much like the flutterings of a butterfly. Second-time mothers often feel the movements sooner, perhaps as early as the fourth month. A woman who is pregnant for the first time may not be aware of her baby's movements until the fifth month.

If your navel is normally regressed, you may find that it begins to push out during this trimester and that it becomes level with the abdomen. You may also notice a dark line beginning to appear down the middle of the abdomen, starting at the navel. This increased pigmentation, like the darkening of the areolae and nipples, is thought to be due to increased hormonal levels. The line will begin to fade sometime after childbirth. By the fifth month, all of the important milk-making structures are fully developed. The breasts, however, will not begin producing milk until after the baby is born. Your breasts will have increased substantially in size, and they may become just a bit fuller during the remaining months of pregnancy.

One more thing that you may notice during this trimester is an increase in body heat. You may find that you perspire more and feel warm even if the weather is moderate.

The Third Trimester

Physical changes during the last months of pregnancy are momentous. The uterus grows increasingly larger and rises higher and higher in the abdominal cavity. As the uterus enlarges, it presses against the bladder and you may again find that you have to urinate more frequently. The enlarging uterus also puts pressure on the pelvic veins, which inhibits the flow of blood from the lower part of the body. This circulatory slowdown can contribute to hemorrhoids and varicose veins, as well as swelling of the legs and ankles. This slowdown is compounded by the fact that blood volume increases by 40 to 90 percent during pregnancy. The increasing weight of the uterus and baby can also contribute to backache and fatigue. As the uterus rises higher in the abdominal cavity, it presses against the stomach, and this can cause or aggravate heartburn. It also causes pressure beneath the diaphragm, and this can lead to shortness of breath. Breathlessness and heartburn are usually relieved when the baby "drops," or becomes engaged.

During this trimester, your nipples may begin to secrete a creamy, yellowish substance. This is colostrum, the forerunner of mature breast milk. If you choose to nurse, colostrum will nourish your baby during the first few days of life. As pregnancy draws to a close, you may also find that your navel protrudes. This can result from the increasing pressure of the expanding uterus. Sometime after birth, the navel will return to its normal position.

From the beginning of this trimester, your doctor or nurse-midwife—and perhaps you also—will be able to identify different parts of the baby's body by feeling your abdomen and will also be able to tell what position the baby is in. During the last month or so of pregnancy, antibodies that you have developed against certain diseases will be passed to your baby via the placenta. These antibodies will help provide her with temporary protection against these diseases after she is born.

During the eighth or ninth month, you will probably experience what are called Braxton Hicks contractions. These contractions actually occur throughout pregnancy, but they become more frequent in the last month or two. Braxton Hicks contractions occur irregularly and are generally painless. Unlike real labor contractions, they will usually subside if you relax. Braxton Hicks contractions do not cause the cervix to dilate or to open and are therefore signs of false labor. Actually, they seem to serve as a rehearsal for labor, helping to prepare the uterus for the work that is to come.

Common Discomforts and How to Relieve Them

As you can see from the above timetable, the bodily changes of pregnancy, while exciting to think about and to watch, can cause some physical discomforts. Each woman, of course, will experience pregnancy differently and may have, in varying degrees, some or all of the discomforts that we will look at. Few women will get through these nine months without feeling at least a little discomfort from fatigue, backache, or breathlessness. On the other hand, very few women will feel terribly uncomfortable throughout pregnancy. Attitude can play a role in how a woman adjusts to the minor complaints of pregnancy. It's true that they can be annoying and uncomfortable, but they are also exciting evidence that a baby is growing inside you. In addition, there are simple measures that you can take to help relieve many of these discomforts if or when they arise.

Nausea

For many women, a queasy stomach is the first sign of pregnancy. While it's commonly called morning sickness, this queasy feeling can occur at any time of the day. It does, however, tend to be worse in the morning because the stomach is empty. As we've seen, it is thought that the hormone HCG contributes to nausea, although exactly how is still not fully understood. What is known

Your Pregnant Body

is that levels of this hormone begin to drop at the end of the first trimester, a time when nausea usually starts to subside and then disappears.

There are a number of things that can be done to help relieve a queasy stomach. If you feel nauseous in the morning, try to start the day more slowly, because an upset stomach can be made worse by a lot of rushing about. Before going to bed at night, leave some dry crackers or cereal on your nightstand. When you wake in the morning, eat the food slowly, then relax in bed for another 15 minutes or so. The crackers or cereal will help absorb stomach acid and get the digestive process going. When you do get up, have a nice leisurely breakfast.

Don't let yourself get hungry during the day, because an empty stomach tends to get upset more easily. Try to eat small, frequent meals, instead of three big ones, which can overload a sensitive stomach. Between meals, snack on protein foods, such as cheese or nuts. It's a good idea also to take liquids separately from meals and to sip them slowly.

Try to avoid very rich, fatty, or spicy foods, as they can often aggravate nausea. Avoid any food whose taste or smell gives you a queasy feeling. During the early months, many women have strong aversions to certain foods, even ones that may have been favorites before pregnancy. Sometimes just the smell of a certain food cooking is enough to set off a wave of nausea. So don't torture yourself, even if a particular food happens to be your husband's favorite.

Fresh air can also help relieve nausea. Be sure your bedroom is well ventilated. In cold weather, give the room a good airing by opening the window for ten or so minutes before you go to bed. If you work outside the home, try to take a walk at lunchtime. When I was pregnant with my son, riding the New York subway at rush hour was sheer agony because of the lack of air. I always felt as if I were suffocating and would become sick to my stomach. The 25-minute ride to work during my first trimester took twice as long, because I had to keep getting off the train to breathe some fresh air and to nibble a cracker.

Finally, never take any medication for nausea without first consulting your physician or nurse-midwife, and this goes for any other discomfort that you may experience during pregnancy. This is not the time for self-medication. You should never take any drug—either prescription or over-the-counter—without your caregiver's knowledge and approval.

Fatigue and Insomnia

The first trimester usually brings an overwhelming feeling of fatigue as the body adjusts to increased hormonal levels. It is not uncommon for a woman to go to bed right after dinner and sleep straight through till morning. Even after this long night's rest, she may still feel tired during the day. The middle months of pregnancy will probably find you revitalized and energetic. As you get into the third trimester, though, the increasing weight of the uterus and baby will be putting new demands on your body, and you will probably find that you are once again pepless and tired. At the same time, you may also be bothered by insomnia. Your body will become increasingly cumbersome, and you may have difficulty finding a comfortable position for sleep. Many babies also perform their wildest gymnastics at night when their moms are trying to get some rest. In addition, you may find yourself waking several times during the night to urinate. Some people say this is nature's way of preparing a mother for the interrupted nights she will have after the baby is born. Actually, it's the enlarging uterus pressing against the bladder. Frequent urination can become even more of a nuisance when the baby "drops," or becomes engaged—that is, when his head or presenting part descends into the pelvis. There are no cures for insomnia. The best thing is to rest and sleep whenever you can during the day. At night, use lots of pillows to support your arms, legs, and stomach, and sleep on your side. Whenever you lie down to rest or sleep during the last three or four months of pregnancy, you should lie on your side and ideally the left side. When you lie on your back, the enlarging uterus can compress major blood vessels, which can result in a dangerous lowering of blood pressure.

Constipation

Some women are troubled with constipation throughout pregnancy; others are never bothered. The increased hormonal levels of the first trimester can contribute to constipation, because they relax the smooth muscle that makes up the intestines. As a result of this relaxation, the bowel is less efficient in getting rid of body wastes. Constipation can be aggravated in the later months as the enlarging uterus crowds the intestines and impedes elimination. One of the best ways to relieve constipation is to eat high-fiber foods—bran, whole grains, raw fruits and vegetables, seeds and nuts. Drinking lots of fluids, especially fruit juices, can also be very helpful, as can getting regular exercise. Iron supplements, which are often prescribed during pregnancy, can aggravate constipation. To help guard against this, it's best to take them at mealtime with a food that is rich in vitamin C, such as grapefruit or orange juice. If constipation is a severe problem for you, discuss it with your doctor or nurse-midwife. Never self-prescribe a laxative, and do not take mineral oil—it interferes with the body's absorption of certain vitamins and minerals.

Heartburn

This annoying discomfort is a type of indigestion and has nothing to do with the heart. It results when stomach acids splash up into the esophagus and cause a burning sensation. Increased hormonal levels can contribute to heartburn, because they relax the smooth sphincter muscle that separates the stomach from the lower end of the esophagus, thus making it easier for gastric juices to be regurgitated. Heartburn can occur at any time during pregnancy, but it is especially common during the later months as the uterus rises in the abdominal cavity and presses against the stomach. The best way to guard against heartburn is to avoid overloading the stomach. As with nausea, eat small, frequent meals throughout the day, and avoid very rich, fatty, or spicy foods. Also resist taking a siesta right after eating, as a reclining position makes it easier for stomach acids to splash back into the esopha-

Your Pregnant Body

gus. Do not take antacids or any other remedy to relieve heartburn without first consulting your physician or nurse-midwife.

Backache

If you experience lower backache in early pregnancy, it will probably be due to the relaxation of the pelvic ligaments, a condition that results when hormonal levels rise. Lower backache usually becomes more of a problem in later pregnancy, because the increasing weight of the baby and uterus tends to pull you forward, which accentuates the natural curve of the spine. The best remedy for backache is to pay close attention to proper posture. Keep your abdominal wall tightened by pulling in and up, and keep your buttocks tucked under; your back should be straight, your shoulders level, and your head erect. Wear shoes with broad, low heels, the lowest heels that are comfortable for you. High heels should be avoided, especially in later pregnancy; they throw the spine out of line and can leave you dangerously off-balance. Also pay close attention to your posture when you are sitting. Sit all the way back in a chair so that your back and shoulders are supported. Keep your feet flat on the floor or rest them on a footstool.

Leg Cramps

These are especially common in the second and third trimesters. They frequently occur at night and may wake you with a start from a sound sleep. It is thought that a calcium-phosphorus imbalance may contribute to leg cramps. Decreased circulation in the lower part of the body may also be a factor. Leg cramps are more likely to strike when you are lying on your back, so try to sleep lying on your side, preferably the left side. You should be doing this in late pregnancy anyway. Leg cramps can be very painful. If one strikes, stretch out your leg, bend your foot upward, and massage the cramped muscle. Repeat this several times or until the cramp disappears. If leg cramps are persistent, speak with your physician or nurse-midwife.

Varicose Veins

The tendency to develop varicose veins is thought to be hereditary, and this condition often appears for the first time during pregnancy. A principal factor in the development of varicose veins is the increased pressure exerted by the enlarging uterus on the pelvic veins, which, in turn, impedes the flow of blood from the lower part of the body. Indeed, varicose veins usually become more and more evident as pregnancy progresses and the uterus becomes increasingly heavy. Preventive measures are the best treatment for varicose veins and should be started early, especially if you have a family history of this condition. Try not to stand for prolonged periods of time, and, whenever possible, lie down and elevate your legs at about a 30-degree angle to the body. Also elevate your legs when you are sitting by propping your feet on a footstool. Regular exercise is also very helpful, especially

Your Pregnant Body

walking, as it helps keep the blood circulating in the legs. Try to take a brisk 20- or 30-minute walk each day. Support panty hose will also help and should be put on first thing in the morning and before you get out of bed. They should be kept on all day and taken off before you retire for the night. If proper precautions are taken during pregnancy, varicose veins often disappear or improve after childbirth.

Hemorrhoids

These are varicose veins of the rectum. Like varicose veins of the legs, hemorrhoids are largely due to the pressure exerted by the expanding uterus on the pelvic veins and the subsequent circulatory slowdown. Hemorrhoids, however, can be aggravated or encouraged by constipation. One of the best preventive measures, therefore, is to keep yourself from getting constipated. Another helpful measure is to avoid straining during bowel movements. Hemorrhoids often become evident during the later months of pregnancy and can be aggravated by the stresses of labor and delivery. In fact, some women only develop hemorrhoids after giving birth. If you develop hemorrhoids, ask your physician or nurse-midwife what she recommends for relieving itching and irritation. Sometimes, applying an ice pack or a witch hazel compress brings relief. Most hemorrhoid problems began to improve after childbirth.

If you experience any of the discomforts that are associated with pregnancy—and you will no doubt experience at least a few—it's important to keep in mind that they are only temporary. Before you know it, they'll be traded in for a new little person. In the meantime, there are many simple measures—from slight adjustments in your eating habits to paying attention to proper posture to elevating your legs—that can help relieve and even help prevent many of these minor discomforts.

The Double-Duty Diet

You are constantly nourishing your baby while you are pregnant. Whatever you eat, he eats. And if you fast, he fasts as well. During these nine months, your baby will need a steady supply of high-quality nutrients and calories to help him grow and develop properly. And you will need the same to help you meet the new demands that pregnancy will place on your body. As important as what you eat is how much you eat. Many studies have shown a direct relationship between maternal weight gain and the baby's weight at birth. And birth weight is a critical factor in how a baby will develop physically and mentally after birth. Eating a well-balanced diet and gaining sufficient weight are two very important things that you can do to help give your baby a good start in life.

Weight Gain: How Much and How Quickly?

Most professionals today recommend an average weight gain of between 24 and 28 pounds. This, of course, is only an average and applies to women whose pre-pregnancy weights are just about right for their heights and body frames. In addition, other factors can influence weight gain. Younger women, for example, tend to gain more

Your Pregnant Body

than older women, and first-time mothers more than second-time mothers. An average gain of between 24 and 28 pounds is considered desirable because a woman is then more likely to give birth to a baby who weighs between 7 and 8 pounds. This, in turn, is considered an optimal

> The average recommended weight gain during pregnancy is between 24 and 28 pounds. This can be accounted for by the following approximations: baby, 7½ pounds; placenta, 1½ pounds; amniotic fluid, 2 pounds; uterus, 2 pounds; increase in breast weight, 1 pound; increase in blood volume, 4 pounds; body fluids and fat stores, 6 to 10 pounds. (Fat stores provide extra energy during pregnancy and help a new mother produce breast milk.)

birth weight. There are, of course, other factors that can influence birth weight. One is the baby's genetic inheritance, which includes the size of his parents. A baby whose parents are slight in build is not likely to be as big as a baby whose parents have medium or large frames. Still, a mother's weight gain is inextricably linked to her baby's birth weight. And statistics clearly show definite advantages for babies who have optimal birth weights. Full-term babies who weigh 7 pounds or more have fewer physical and mental handicaps, are less susceptible to serious illnesses, and have a lower infant mortality rate than full-term babies who weigh 5½ pounds or less. Five and a half pounds is generally considered to be the lowest adequate birth weight, but a much higher weight than this is desirable. A baby's physical and mental health, of course, is influenced by other factors besides birth weight. We have little or no control over some of these, such as genetic and environmental influences. We do, however, have control over what and how much we eat.

A woman who begins pregnancy underweight should have a higher than average weight gain. Most professionals recommend that she gain between 24 and 28 pounds plus the number of pounds she lacked before pregnancy according to average standards for her height and body frame. Good weight gain is very important for an underweight woman. If she fails to gain sufficient weight, she is at greater risk of having a low-weight baby and of developing toxemia, a serious condition of pregnancy.

A woman who is overweight when she becomes pregnant may have a slightly lower than average weight gain. Recommendations often range from 18 to 24 pounds, and some professionals believe that an overweight woman should follow the same recommended weight gain of 24 to 28 pounds that is made for a woman of normal weight. Pregnancy is *not* a time to try to lose weight. Rather, it is a time to pay close attention to the quality of foods that are eaten. People who are obese are often undernourished, because much of the weight is usually the result of consuming a lot of "junk" foods, instead of foods that are rich in protein, vitamins, and minerals. An expectant mother who is overweight needs to improve her eating habits so the emphasis is on quality and not empty-calorie foods. No expectant mother, whatever her weight, should try to diet or skip meals. Remember, the growing baby needs a steady supply of high-quality nutrients and calories to help him grow and develop properly.

It's important to keep in mind that your *rate* of weight gain is as important as the *amount* of weight gain. During the first trimester, you should expect to gain between 2 and 4 pounds. After that, you should gain about 1 pound a week. A steadily increasing gain is what is desirable. Any rapid gain—2 or 3 or more pounds within a week—should be reported to your physician or nurse-midwife. A sudden jump in weight can be an indication of toxemia. In the case of toxemia, weight gain is due to an accumulation of excess water, not to healthy tissue and fat stores.

You should also keep in mind that much of the weight that you gain during pregnancy will be lost within a few weeks after birth. Just the baby, placenta, and amniotic fluid may account for 11 to 13 pounds—and this weight is lost immediately after delivery. With attention to exercise and sound nutrition, most new mothers find that they're back to pre-pregnancy form by three to six months after birth.

What and How Much Should You Eat?

To achieve an adequate weight gain, the average expectant mother must increase her caloric intake by at least 300 calories a day and even more if she is active. The quality of the food that you eat is just as important as the quantity. More than ever, you need to eat a well-balanced diet drawn from the four basic food groups: protein foods, milk and dairy products, fruits and vegetables, and grains. This is the only way other than supplementation that you can get the nutrients that are necessary to help keep you healthy and to help make a healthy baby. You need protein, carbohydrates, fats, vitamins, and minerals to do that.

Protein Foods Protein is an essential component of body cells. Since an expectant mother is helping to build a whole new person who is made up of cells, her protein requirement is greatly increased, and she needs about two-thirds more each day. Protein foods include meat, fish, poultry, eggs, and dried beans and peas (soybeans, kidney beans, lentils, etc.). To help you meet your increased need for protein, you should have at least three servings each day from this group.

Proteins are composed of amino acids. Animal proteins are complete because they contain all the essential amino acids. Plant proteins are either low or lacking in one or two and so are incomplete. If you are a vegetarian, you are probably knowledgeable about combining different foods to form a proper balance of all essential amino acids—dried beans and rice, for example. Pregnancy, however, calls for unique nutritional needs, and it would be wise to get professional assistance with diet planning to be sure that your baby is receiving all the nutrients that he needs for proper growth and development. This is especially important if you do not consume any animal proteins, including dairy products and eggs. If you do not know a registered dietician who has expertise in this area, your physician or nurse-midwife should be able to refer you to one.

Milk and Dairy Products These are good sources of protein, and they are the best sources of calcium and phosphorus, which are essential in building your baby's bones and teeth. These two minerals are so important during pregnancy that your need for them increases one and a half times. The best way to assure that you get enough of each is to drink 1 quart of milk each day. If you dislike drinking milk straight from the glass, you may find it more tolerable when it's combined with cereal, or when it's used in soups, puddings, and casseroles. You can also use other dairy products as substitutes. For example, 1 cup of yogurt, 1½ cups of cottage cheese, and 1½ ounces of hard cheese such as Swiss or cheddar each supply the equivalent of 1 cup of milk. Fortified whole milk is also an excellent source of vitamin D, which helps the body use calcium and phosphorus efficiently. One quart of fortified whole milk will satisfy your daily requirement for vitamin D, as well as for calcium and phosphorus.

Fruits and Vegetables You should have at least four servings of fruits and vegetables each day. They are excellent sources of vitamins (especially A and C), trace minerals, and fiber. Fresh fruits also provide carbohydrates, which are essential during pregnancy. You should have one to two servings of citrus fruit, which is rich in vitamin C; two servings of leafy green, yellow, or orange vegetables, which are excellent sources of vitamin A; then at least one more serving of another fruit or vegetable.

Grains This group includes breads, cereals, pastas, rice, and wheat germ. Grain products are an important source of carbohydrates, and you should have at least four servings each day. Try to choose whole-grain products. They're a good source of fiber, certain B vitamins, and trace minerals and are generally more nourishing than products made from processed and refined grains. Do *not* skimp on grain products during pregnancy. They are a major source of carbohydrates, which provide fuel for the body. You need a steady supply of this fuel and so does your baby. Remember, too, that fresh fruits are also good sources of wholesome carbohydrates.

Liquids You should also drink plenty of liquids during

pregnancy—at least a quart in addition to milk. Water is an excellent choice, and so are fruit and vegetable juices. Avoid soft drinks and beverages that contain caffeine, such as cola, tea, and coffee (more about caffeine on page 85). Extra liquids will help prevent constipation, and they're needed to help maintain your expanded blood volume and the increased amount of body fluids.

Your Daily Diet

Food Group	Servings	Equivalent of One Serving
Protein Foods	3+	3 oz. lean cooked meat, poultry, or fish; 2 eggs; 1 cup cooked dried beans or peas, such as soybeans, kidney beans, garbanzo beans, lentils, blackeye peas, split peas
Milk and Dairy Products	4	1 cup milk; 1 cup yogurt; 1½ oz. hard cheese, such as Swiss or cheddar; 1½ cups cottage cheese
Fruits and Vegetables	4+*	1 orange; ½ grapefruit; 1 cup raw or ¾ cup cooked spinach, kale, carrots, sweet potato, broccoli, Brussels sprouts, winter squash; 1 potato; 1 apple; ½ cantaloupe
Grains	4+	1 slice bread; ¾ to 1 cup ready-to-eat cereal; ½ to ¾ cup cooked cereal; ½ to ¾ cup rice or pasta; ¼ cup wheat germ
Liquids	4 to 6	1 cup water or fruit or vegetable juice

*(1 to 2 servings citrus fruit; 2 servings leafy green, yellow, or orange vegetables; at least 1 more serving other vegetable or fruit)

Other Nutritional Needs

Iron and Folic Acid Increased caloric intake and a well-balanced diet can satisfy nearly all of the extra nutritional

Your Pregnant Body

needs of pregnancy. There are, however, two exceptions: iron and, to a lesser extent, folic acid or folacin, which is one of the B vitamins.

The body's need for iron doubles during pregnancy, and it is usually not possible to meet this new demand through diet alone. As a result, iron supplements are generally prescribed during the second and third trimesters. Iron is vital to the development of red blood cells. Since a woman's blood volume can increase by 40 to 90 percent during pregnancy, you can easily see why extra iron is needed. Red blood cells, in turn, carry oxygen not only throughout the mother's body but to the placenta and the baby. During the last trimester, too, the baby begins to store iron for use after birth, and this further taxes the mother's own supply.

Even if iron supplements are prescribed, a woman should still eat iron-rich foods. These include liver, kidney, egg yolk, dried beans, leafy green vegetables (such as spinach and kale), and raisins and dried fruits, which, by the way, make wholesome snacks. Iron supplements can make one constipated, and it's best to take them with a vitamin C food, such as orange or grapefruit juice. This will help the iron be better absorbed by the body.

In addition to iron, supplements are often prescribed for folic acid or folacin. The need for this B vitamin doubles during pregnancy, and, like iron, it is often not possible to meet this new demand through diet alone. Folic acid is essential in the process of cell division. Since an expectant mother is helping to build a whole new person who is made up of cells, it is easy to understand why this vitamin is so vital. Folic acid also enables red blood cells to carry oxygen throughout the mother's body and to the placenta and baby. Like iron, folic acid supplements are usually prescribed during the second and third trimesters, but even if they are prescribed, a woman should still eat foods that are good sources of this vitamin. These include liver, kidney, leafy green vegetables, dried beans, and wheat germ. As you can see, these are many of the foods that are also rich in iron, so when you eat them, you are helping to meet two important nutritional needs, as well as many others.

Multivitamin-Mineral Supplements With the exceptions of iron and folic acid, the extra nutritional needs of pregnancy can usually be satisfied by eating a well-balanced diet. Many caregivers, however, prescribe a multivitamin-mineral supplement as a precautionary measure. You should, by the way, *never* take any vitamin or mineral supplement on your own. Excessive doses of certain vitamins can be toxic and harmful to the baby (more about this in the next section). Even when multivitamin-mineral supplements are prescribed, they are not intended to take the place of sound nutrition, and no caregiver prescribes them for that purpose. They are viewed only as extra insurance that a woman will have enough of the essential vitamins and minerals that she and her baby need. There is virtual agreement that the best way a mother can help assure her health and her baby's is to increase her caloric intake and eat a well-balanced diet drawn from the four basic food groups. What a tasty insurance policy that is!

Drugs and the Unborn Baby

Not so very long ago, it was thought that the placenta served as a barrier. Somehow it filtered out most harmful substances but allowed oxygen and nutrients to be passed to the baby. Today, however, we know that the placenta's role as a barrier is virtually nonexistent and that any substance taken by the mother can reach the baby. It was the thalidomide tragedy of the early 1960s that made this perfectly clear and that led to a greater awareness of the potential risks that drugs pose to the unborn baby.

Thalidomide was a tranquilizer that was marketed in England and West Germany but not in the United States, where it still had not been approved by the FDA. It had undergone a variety of tests and appeared to be effective and safe. Shortly after it was introduced, however, physicians began noting an increase in the number of babies being born with a rare malformation of the arms and legs. In follow-up investigations, it was learned that in nearly every case, the mother had taken thalidomide in early pregnancy.

While much progress has been made during the past 20 years in understanding the relationship between drugs and birth defects, there is still insufficient information on the possible effects most drugs can have on the unborn baby. No drug, however, has been proven to be 100 percent safe, and whenever a medication is prescribed during pregnancy, the benefits must be carefully weighed against the risks. The prudent thing is to avoid all medication unless it is absolutely necessary for your health or the health of your baby. It is also important to keep things in perspective. Approximately 2 percent of all babies are born with major birth defects, and 5 to 10 percent of these can thus far be attributed to teratogens, which are environmental hazards including drugs. About 65 percent of birth defects are still of unknown origin. While the risk of such defects may seem relatively small, it is a risk that can be easily avoided.

Researchers generally believe that most birth defects are the result of a combination of factors, particularly the interaction of an environmental hazard, or teratogen, and an inherited susceptibility in the unborn baby. This would explain why some babies who were exposed to thalidomide did not develop malformations. Timing, or when a drug is taken during pregnancy, is also a critical factor. The baby is most vulnerable to chemical agents during the first trimester and especially during the first two months. This is when the baby's internal organs and systems are developing. It is during this time of rapid cell division that drugs and other teratogens can have the most damaging effect. During the second and third trimesters, the risk of major deformities is less. Drugs, however, can continue to pose a risk to the baby's proper growth and development. Tetracycline, for example, can retard bone growth and discolor the baby's teeth. Iodide compounds, which are used to treat asthma, can result in the formation of fetal goiters. Another critical factor is dosage—how much of a drug is taken and for how long. The higher the dose and the longer it is taken, the greater the potential risk.

There are, of course, situations in which medications

must be taken. Certain maternal illnesses, such as epilepsy, can pose a serious threat to the unborn baby if left untreated. Ideally, a woman who has a serious medical condition—such as epilepsy, heart disease, thyroid disorders, and chronic asthma—should get professional advice about medications before she becomes pregnant. Even in a low-risk pregnancy, a condition may arise where the benefits of taking a drug would outweigh the potential risks—a urinary tract infection, for example, which can be treated with an antibiotic that has been found to be relatively safe. But no drug should be taken during pregnancy unless it is absolutely essential to either your health or your baby's, and you should never take any medication without first consulting your physician or nurse-midwife. Pregnancy is not the time to self-medicate. If a drug is prescribed for you, you should ask about its safety and the possible risks to the baby. Individual illnesses can often be treated with a variety of drugs, and your caregiver should be able to choose a medication that offers the greatest benefit with the least risk. And he should be willing to discuss the pros and cons of different drugs with you so that you are completely informed. If you wish, you can check on the relative safety of various medications yourself by consulting a copy of *Physicians' Desk Reference*, which should be available in your local library.

Over-the-Counter Drugs

The rule about not self-medicating during pregnancy applies to over-the-counter drugs as well as to prescription drugs. Actually, medicines and remedies that can be purchased without a prescription may pose a greater risk than prescription drugs, because they are so accessible and so little understood by the average consumer. Advertising has induced us to be a very drug-oriented society, and most of us reach for an aspirin tablet or a cold pill as easily as we reach for a bite to eat. But over-the-counter medicines are not necessarily safe for you and your baby just because you do not need a prescription to get them. Some of them, in fact, are definitely known to be harmful, especially when taken in large doses.

Aspirin is a case in point. When it is taken in large amounts during the last months of pregnancy, it may cause bleeding disorders in both the baby and the mother. Heavy consumption in the last trimester has also been associated with prolonging the length of pregnancy and of labor. There is also some evidence that high doses of aspirin in early pregnancy may be linked to fetal malformations, although the evidence on this is still considered circumstantial. But it isn't enough to avoid taking just aspirin during pregnancy. Scores of over-the-counter products contain aspirin. Virtually all pain relief preparations (except acetaminophen compounds, such as Tylenol®) contain aspirin, as do many cold remedies. Some over-the-counter antacids contain sodium bicarbonate, which can cause edema, or swelling, due to fluid retention. Many nonprescription sleep aids contain the antihistamine pyrilamine. While no known ill-effects have thus far been reported, it is certainly prudent not to use any over-the-counter sleep aids during pregnancy. The bottom line is: Do not use any over-the-counter medication— whether it be for a headache, a cold, an allergy, an upset stomach, heartburn, or constipation—without first consulting your physician or nurse-midwife.

Caffeine

You may not think of caffeine as a drug, but it affects your body and your baby's as if it were. Caffeine stimulates the central nervous system and can cause irritability, anxiety, insomnia, and disturbances in the heart rate and rhythm. More importantly, caffeine can freely cross the placenta and enter the baby's bloodstream, which is why you should be very wary of it during pregnancy.

At the present time, there is no conclusive evidence that caffeine has ever caused birth defects in human beings. However, laboratory studies have shown that high levels of caffeine fed to pregnant rats caused birth defects in their offspring. The results of these tests have prompted the FDA to issue an advisory to pregnant women to avoid or to use very sparingly foods and drugs that contain caffeine.

Caffeine is found not only in coffee and tea, but also in cocoa, chocolate, cola drinks, and some other soft drinks too. In addition, caffeine is used in literally thousands of prescription and over-the-counter drugs, from pain relievers to cold remedies to stay-awake products. Which is all the more reason not to self-medicate. Until the verdict comes in on caffeine, it is certainly prudent to cut down if not completely eliminate your consumption of products that contain caffeine. Decaffeinated coffee is an alternative, or you might want to try grain-based coffees. Instead of soft drinks, stick with fruit and vegetables juices. They're a lot healthier and satisfy thirst just as well as soda pop—maybe even better.

Vitamin and Mineral Supplements

One common but inaccurate assumption that we often make is that if something is good for us, more of it must be better. In many cases, this simply is not true. It definitely is not true in the cases of vitamins A and D. Yes, there are certain daily requirements for these vitamins, and they generally can be met through eating a well-balanced diet. Excessive doses of vitamins A and D, however, can be toxic and can adversely affect the fetus. Excessive amounts of vitamin C may also pose a risk. It is thought that if a woman takes high doses of this vitamin during pregnancy, it may possibly cause scurvy in the newborn, because he is suddenly deprived of the accustomed amounts. You should never take any vitamin or mineral supplements during pregnancy that have not been prescribed by your physician or nurse-midwife. And for those that are, you should never take more than the recommended daily dose.

Sound Reason Not to Smoke

According to the American Cancer Society, 28.9 percent of American women smoke cigarettes. So if you smoke, you are not alone. If you continue to smoke while you are pregnant, however, you should be aware that when you smoke, so does your baby. Whatever you inhale is absorbed into your bloodstream and will eventually cross the placenta, with potentially harmful results. There is now abundant evidence linking cigarette smoking to a range of disorders affecting both the fetus and the newborn baby. And the chances of problems developing increase sharply not only with smoking but with the number of cigarettes a woman smokes each day.

The relationship between smoking and lower birth weight is the most well established of all. Women who smoke during pregnancy tend to have babies who weigh less than babies born to women who do not smoke—on the average about ½ pound lighter. In addition, the babies tend to be shorter in length and to have smaller head circumferences. The relationship between smoking and lower birth weight is independent of all other factors that can influence birth weight. Let's say that two women of equal height and body frame begin pregnancy at the same weight. They both have normal pregnancies, eat well-balanced diets, and they each gain 28 pounds. The only difference is that one woman smokes and the other doesn't. Statistics clearly show that the woman who smokes will have a baby who weighs less than the woman who does not smoke. What's more, birth weight is in proportion to the number of cigarettes that are smoked. Put another way, as the number of cigarettes increases, birth weight decreases. Compared to nonsmokers, the chance of giving birth to a low-weight baby or one who weighs 5½ pounds or less is about 70 percent higher for women who smoke a pack or less of cigarettes each day. For women who smoke a pack or more, it is about 160 percent higher. Remember, between 7 and 8 pounds is considered an optimal birth weight for a baby. Babies who weigh 5½ pounds or less, when compared with babies who weigh 7 pounds or more, have more mental and physical handicaps, as well as a higher mortality rate.

Lower birth weight is not the only problem associated with smoking during pregnancy. It has also been linked to an increased risk of miscarriage, premature delivery, and stillbirth. In addition, some studies have found a higher incidence of hyperactivity and learning disabilities among children whose mothers smoked during pregnancy, as well as slightly lower IQs. Smoking may also increase the risk of certain complications for the mother. Abnormalities of the placenta, particularly placenta previa and abruptio placenta, are much more common in women who smoke than in women who don't. As with lower birth weight, these risks appear to be dose-related. In other words, the more a woman smokes during pregnancy, the greater the risk.

Cigarette smoke contains many harmful substances, but nicotine and especially carbon monoxide are thought to be the most detrimental to the fetus. Both of these substances are absorbed into the mother's bloodstream and readily cross the placenta, and both of them are responsible for decreasing the baby's oxygen supply. Studies have shown a significant reduction in fetal breathing soon after a mother smokes a cigarette, and it may take more than an hour before the breathing pattern becomes normal again. When the fetus does not get enough oxygen, the result is a retardation of growth.

If you smoke, the kindest thing that you can do for your baby and yourself is to stop. If you've previously worried about gaining weight when quitting, pregnancy can be the perfect time for you to stop. After all, you're supposed to gain weight now. And while taking care of yourself may not have been adequate incentive for you before, your feelings of love and responsibility for another life may be just the push you need. When you quit, put away some or all of the money you'll be saving on cigarettes for something either for yourself or for the baby.

If you need help in quitting, there are a number of programs available for smokers who want to stop. Contact the American Cancer Society, the American Lung Association, or the American Heart Association for information. Your physician or nurse-midwife should also be knowledgeable about such programs in the community. Remember, it is not too late to quit. Ideally, a woman should stop smoking before she becomes pregnant, but even if she stops by the fourth month, studies indicate that some of the harmful effects of smoking can be ameliorated, especially the most common problem—a lower birth-weight baby.

Why Alcohol and Pregnancy Don't Mix

Alcohol readily crosses the placenta and enters the baby's bloodstream in the same concentration as in the mother's. When a woman becomes intoxicated, so does her baby.

A women who drinks six or more alcoholic beverages a day is at high risk of giving birth to a baby with Fetal Alcohol Syndrome (FAS). A baby born with FAS is malnourished, underweight, and often mentally retarded, has head and facial abnormalities, and may have heart and limb deformities as well. Although it is not known exactly how the abnormalities are caused, or why FAS occurs in some babies born to women who are heavy drinkers and not in others, the connection with alcohol is clear. Even more moderate drinking can be potentially harmful. Women who have two or more drinks a day tend to have babies who weigh less than babies of women who drink infrequently or not at all. There is also evidence that binge drinking is harmful and should be avoided. Any large doses of alcohol, even occasional ones, can be risky. The period of greatest vulnerability is immediately after conception and during the early months of pregnancy when the baby's organs are forming, and also in late pregnancy when the brain is undergoing accelerated development.

The effect alcohol can have on the unborn baby is a relatively new area of investigation. While it is known that heavy drinking poses a definite threat to the unborn baby, it is still not clear what effect light and occasional drinking may have. There are many questions that remain to be answered, and until all the facts are known, the prudent thing is to exercise extreme caution. The Surgeon General advises that the best precaution is not to drink at all if you are considering becoming pregnant or if you are already pregnant. And most researchers concur that abstinence is the wisest course to follow.

Prenatal Care

Like eating well and avoiding harmful substances, getting regular prenatal care is an integral part of your insurance of having a healthy baby—and for your baby to

Your Pregnant Body

have a healthy mother. The majority of pregnancies are uncomplicated, and yours will undoubtedly be one of them, but the examinations and routine tests performed by your caregiver will allow him to detect and treat any problems that might arise while they are still minor.

Many women look forward to their prenatal appointments for the reassurance they provide that everything is normal and for the additional information that is gleaned about the baby. "I've never liked going to doctors and always put off seeing one unless it is absolutely necessary for an illness," says one expectant mother. "But I find I can hardly wait the four weeks between appointments with my obstetrician. It's exciting to be told how the baby is growing, to listen to the heartbeat. The visits also make me feel as if I'm doing something, that time is passing."

Caregivers vary somewhat in how frequently they want to see their expecting patients. In general, prenatal appointments are scheduled for every four weeks until the 28th week of pregnancy, every two to three weeks until the 36th week, and every week after that until delivery. If any problems should develop along the way or if your pregnancy is determined to be high-risk, your caregiver may want to see you more frequently.

The First Prenatal Visit

Quite a bit of time is usually allotted for the first prenatal visit, which is an important one. A detailed medical history will be taken, including information about your menstrual cycle; about any existing medical conditions; and about any previous illnesses, operations, pregnancies, miscarriages, and abortions. All of this information is essential, as it helps alert your caregiver to possible problems. In addition to your medical history, a family medical history will be taken. This will help your caregiver determine if you have any predisposition to multiple births, genetic disorders, or diseases such as diabetes. Your caregiver should also discuss proper nutrition and adequate weight gain, as well as the type of work you do and whether it might have any effect on your pregnancy.

A thorough physical examination, including a pelvic exam, will also be done during the first prenatal visit. Your weight and height will be recorded, and your caregiver will check your skin color, which is an indication of general health, and carefully examine your neck for possible swollen glands. She will listen to your heart and lungs with a stethoscope and examine your breasts and abdomen. The reason for this thorough going-over is to be sure that you are in good health at the start of pregnancy. During the pelvic exam, your caregiver will check the condition of the cervix and the size of the uterus. The size of the bony pelvis will also be checked, although it is still too early to determine if it is adequate to allow for the baby's passage. This can be done toward the end of pregnancy, when your caregiver has a better idea of how large your baby is.

In addition to the physical exam and the medical histories, a number of routine lab tests form an integral part of the first prenatal visit. These screening procedures usually include the following:

Urinalysis You will be asked for a urine sample, which will be tested for the presence of any infections. Urinary tract infections are common during pregnancy but are not always noticeable to the mother. They should, however, be treated promptly. The urine will also be tested for the presence of sugar (glucose) and protein (albumin). Sugar in the urine can be an indication of diabetes. Some women develop diabetes only during pregnancy, and this is called gestational diabetes. If sugar is found in the urine or if a woman has a family history of diabetes, a glucose tolerance test will be done. Protein in the urine can be a sign of toxemia, which is a serious condition of pregnancy. Another indication of toxemia is elevated blood pressure, and this is one reason why your blood pressure will be recorded at each prenatal visit, including the first. Toxemia is discussed later in this section, on pages 102 to 103.

Blood Type and Rh Factor A blood sample will be taken and will provide a great deal of important information. Your blood will be typed to see if you belong to the A, B, AB, or O blood group, and your Rh factor (whether you are positive or negative) will be determined. This information is essential in case a blood transfusion ever becomes necessary. The Rh factor is vital for another reason too. If a woman is Rh negative, her baby may be at risk for developing Rh disease, although this is less likely to happen in a first pregnancy than in a subsequent pregnancy. Rh disease is discussed on pages 100 to 101. Thanks to medical advances, it is far less common today than in the past.

Blood Count A complete count will also be done to determine if you are anemic. Anemia is common during pregnancy and is usually due to iron deficiency. As we've seen, iron is vital to the development of red blood cells, which, in turn, carry oxygen throughout the mother's body and to the baby. It is essential that anemia be controlled so that neither the mother nor the baby is deprived of sufficient oxygen. In most cases, anemia can be kept in check with iron supplements.

Rubella Your blood will also be screened for the presence of rubella or German measles antibodies, whether or not you have had this disease. It is possible that if you had a very mild case, your body did not produce sufficient antibodies to protect you from contracting the disease again. If this is so, or if you have never had rubella or were not vaccinated against it before you became pregnant, you should stay away from anyone who has it. If an expectant mother contracts rubella, it poses a very serious danger to the baby, especially if she gets the disease during the first trimester. A woman should never be vaccinated against rubella if she suspects that she is pregnant.

STDs This stands for sexually transmitted diseases, which include syphilis, gonorrhea, and venereal herpes. A blood test is used to screen for syphilis, and in most states, this test during pregnancy is required by law. Of the sexually transmitted diseases, syphilis is the most devastating and the one that poses the greatest danger to the baby before birth. The syphilis spirochete crosses the placenta and can lead to miscarriage, stillbirth, or a baby who is born with the disease. Infection of the newborn is called congenital syphilis, and it can be active or latent. Congenital syphilis is usually contracted during the last five months of pregnancy. To help guard against this, it is vital that syphilis be diagnosed early in pregnancy so that appropriate antibiotic treatment can be started. If syphilis is detected early and promptly treated, the baby has a good chance of being born healthy.

Gonorrhea poses the biggest threat to the baby at the time of delivery. If his mother has an active infection, it can be transmitted to the baby during his passage through the birth canal. The biggest danger is to the baby's eyes. They may become infected by the gonorrhea bacterium, and this, in turn, can lead to partial or complete blindness. This is why prophylactic drops are routinely put in the eyes of newborns shortly after birth. Gonorrhea can be diagnosed by taking a cervical smear and having it cultivated, and many caregivers do this screening procedure routinely during the first prenatal visit. If gonorrhea is detected, it can be treated with appropriate antibiotics.

At the present time, there is no cure for venereal herpes or herpes simplex virus II. Venereal herpes is the most active venereal disease in the United States today and is characterized by blisters or sores, together with fever and pain. The sores are most frequently in the genital area but can appear on other parts of the body too. Venereal herpes poses the biggest threat to the baby at the time of delivery. An active infection on the mother's cervix, vagina, or vulva can be transmitted to the baby and can lead to neurological damage and even death. Women who have a history of venereal herpes, and also women who don't, will be carefully watched throughout pregnancy for signs of the disease. If suspicious sores develop, a culture can be taken for diagnosis. A woman who has an active infection in the last weeks of pregnancy should not deliver vaginally. Cesarean section is the safest route for the baby.

Pap Smear This routine test for cervical cancer is usually included in the first prenatal checkup, especially if it has not been recently done.

As you can see, the first prenatal visit is lengthy and provides a lot of important medical information. But it is important from a personal standpoint too. This is really the first opportunity, other than your preliminary consultation, for you to get a feel for the caregiver you've chosen. Is she attentive, gentle, and thorough? Does she answer your questions thoughtfully and clearly? Or is she the opposite—impatient, dogmatic, and abrupt? If you are satisfied with this first visit, you have reason to feel confident about your future relationship with your caregiver. If you are not satisfied, you may want to think about changing caregivers.

Subsequent Visits

The rest of your prenatal visits will be relatively short and uneventful, unless a complication develops. During each visit, you will be weighed, your blood pressure will be recorded, and a urine sample will be taken. Weight gain provides an important indication of how the baby is developing. A steady weight gain during the second and third trimesters is a good sign. If a woman does not gain sufficient weight or if she loses weight, her baby may not be growing and developing properly. The baby's growth can also be estimated by palpating, or feeling, the abdomen, and your caregiver will do this during each prenatal visit. Urinalysis is done routinely, to ensure that you are not developing an infection, gestational diabetes, or toxemia. A rapid weight gain or a rise in blood pressure can also indicate toxemia. During the third trimester, the blood test for syphilis may be repeated and at about 32 weeks, another complete blood count may be done to check for anemia. As your due date approaches and you are seeing your caregiver once a week, a pelvic exam will be done during each visit. This will let your caregiver determine whether the cervix is beginning to efface and dilate—that is, to thin and open. During the last weeks, cervical cultures may be done for gonorrhea and venereal herpes. Many caregivers do this routinely.

At about 20 weeks, your caregiver will try to detect your baby's heartbeat with a fetoscope. Some caregivers try sooner and may or may not be successful. Not hearing the heartbeat early on does not mean there is something wrong with the baby. It simply means that the baby is still too small or is in a position that makes the heartbeat difficult to detect.

Hearing the heartbeat is a momentous occasion. It gives you a sense, perhaps for the first time, of the baby's reality. This is especially true if you hear the heartbeat before you feel the baby move. It's especially exciting to share this occasion with your spouse. Ask your caregiver when he plans to listen for the heartbeat, then try to schedule it so your husband can be there too. "Hearing the heartbeat was so special," says one expectant mother, "and it was perfect having my husband there. Neither of us expected to be so overcome with emotion, but when we heard that galloping sound, we held hands and grinned from ear to ear. I know a few tears escaped from my eyes. I'm not sure about my husband. But if he didn't cry, I know he felt like it inside."

If for some reason your husband can't be present when

you first hear your baby's heartbeat, you should try to have him come to at least one of the prenatal visits. It will give him a chance to get to know the caregiver, to ask questions, and to learn more about the pregnancy. Your husband (or you, perhaps) may feel that it isn't important for him to come to an appointment, but he may change his mind once he gets there. Says an expectant mother: "My husband agreed to come, but I think he felt very silly about it—especially sitting in the waiting room with all those women. He said he'd just watch, that he had nothing to say. But when we got into the doctor's office, he had lots of questions. I guess he'd been thinking about a lot of things and hadn't even realized it. We were both very glad that he had come."

As your due date approaches, your caregiver should give you guidelines about how to know you are in labor and when to call him. If he doesn't, be sure to initiate the discussion yourself. You should also use your last prenatal appointments to review with your caregiver the type of birth experience you would like to have.

Warning Signs

Any potential problems are usually detected during prenatal visits. Occasionally, however, a problem may arise between appointments. The following are signs that something may be wrong. If you experience any of them, call your caregiver promptly.

1. Vaginal bleeding: Many expectant mothers experience some bleeding, and most of them go on to have normal

pregnancies and healthy babies. Spotting or bleeding, however, should *not* be ignored. It could indicate a threatened miscarriage or a problem with the placenta. Call your caregiver.

2. Abdominal pain: Some aches and pains are to be expected during pregnancy. Abdominal pain that is severe and persistent, however, may mean that something is wrong with the placenta or that another abdominal emergency exists, such as ectopic pregnancy. This means that the fertilized egg has implanted outside the uterus, most often in a Fallopian tube. An ectopic pregnancy cannot develop normally, and if the condition goes undetected, the growing embryo can strain the tube and cause it to burst. This is an emergency situation.

3. Blurred vision and severe, persistent headache: Either of these can be signs of toxemia. Do not ignore them.

4. Vaginal discharge: An increase in vaginal discharge is normal during pregnancy, but if it changes color or has an unpleasant odor, you may have an infection. If the discharge appears to be clear fluid, call your caregiver promptly. There may be a leak in the amniotic sac.

5. Severe vomiting: Nausea and some vomiting are common during the first trimester, but severe vomiting at any time during pregnancy should be reported to your caregiver.

6. Fever: If you have a fever of 100°F or above, you may have an infection that should be treated. High maternal fevers also pose a risk to the fetus, especially in the early months of pregnancy.

Complications

While the majority of pregnancies are normal and medically uneventful, complications do arise for some women. With early detection and proper treatment, however, many of them can be successfully managed. The following are some of the more common complications of pregnancy:

Rh Disease

The Rh factor is a substance on the surface of blood cells. About 85 percent of the world's population has this factor and their blood is Rh positive. People who lack the Rh factor are Rh negative. There is nothing wrong with Rh negative blood. During pregnancy, however, there is a potential problem if the mother is Rh negative and the baby is Rh positive. If positive cells from the baby enter the mother's bloodstream, her body will react by forming antibodies that will attack her baby's blood. Although the circulatory systems of the mother and baby are completely separate, blood cells may occasionally leak from the baby to the mother. Such a leakage is most likely to occur during delivery. If this is the woman's first pregnancy and birth, her baby is not likely to be affected because he is born before antibodies form. To help safeguard a subsequent pregnancy, the mother is given a vaccine called RhoGAM within 72 hours after delivery. RhoGAM usually destroys the positive cells before the mother's body has time to develop antibodies or become sensitized. Without RhoGAM, the antibodies would become a permanent part of her bloodstream and would pose a potential threat to her next pregnancy. A woman with Rh negative blood should be given RhoGAM after each delivery of an Rh positive baby, and also after other situations that could cause sensitization, including a miscarriage, abortion, and an ectopic pregnancy. Through oversight or carelessness, however, this may not always be done, and it is essential that an expectant mother tell her caregiver about any situation in which she might have been exposed to Rh positive blood, including blood transfusions.

The routine blood test that is done at the first prenatal visit for blood type and Rh factor also screens for antibodies. If no antibodies are detected in an Rh negative mother, another blood test will be done later, usually at the 24th week and again at the 32nd. In a first pregnancy, remember, it is not likely that antibodies will develop until after delivery, and these subsequent blood tests are mainly precautionary measures. If for some reason an Rh negative mother has become sensitized and antibodies are detected with the first blood test, she will be carefully monitored throughout pregnancy. Blood tests will probably be done every four to six weeks to determine the level of antibodies. If a critical level is reached, additional diagnostic testing, including ultrasound and amniocentesis, will be done to evaluate the baby's condition. If he is in danger, he may be given a blood transfusion while he is in the uterus, or he may be delivered early and, if necessary, given a blood-exchange transfusion. Fortunately, Rh disease is not as common as it once was, thanks to RhoGAM.

Toxemia

This is a serious condition of pregnancy, and if it occurs, it usually develops in the last trimester, although it can occur earlier. Toxemia is divided into two stages—preeclampsia and eclampsia. Preeclampsia is characterized by the three symptoms: elevated blood pressure, protein in the urine, and edema, which is swelling due to water retention. Some amount of swelling is common during pregnancy, especially of the legs and feet. Swelling of the face and fingers is more characteristic of toxemia. Remember, if you have a sudden weight gain—2 or 3 or more pounds within a week—you should call your caregiver. If the weight is due to fluid retention, it could be a sign of toxemia. Preeclampsia is usually managed with rest and special attention to proper nutrition. It is vital that preeclampsia be kept under control so that it does not develop into eclampsia, which is characterized by convulsion and possibly coma. With proper management and treatment, most cases of toxemia never reach this stage. Warning signs of an advancing case of toxemia include rapidly rising blood pressure, a severe, persistent headache, blurred vision, irritability, and stomach pain. In cases of advancing toxemia, a woman will be hospitalized to keep the condition from worsening and leading to eclampsia or, in other words, a dangerous convulsion. The baby's maturity will be evaluated, and if the pregnancy is close to term, labor will probably be induced.

Exactly what causes toxemia is not known. Some evidence suggests that it may be due to a decrease in the blood supply to the uterus. Toxemia occurs most frequently in first pregnancies and in multiple pregnancies. Women with diabetes and kidney disease are also at greater risk, as are those with a history of high blood pressure. After delivery, the condition disappears.

Placenta Previa

This is a condition in which the placenta partially or totally covers the cervix. Normally, the placenta implants high in the uterus; if it implants too low, placenta previa can result. Bleeding is usually the only sign of placenta previa—there is no pain associated with it. Any spotting or bleeding, of course, should be reported promptly to your caregiver. If placenta previa is suspected, it can be best diagnosed with ultrasound. Women with placenta previa usually bleed intermittently during pregnancy, and with each episode, the bleeding typically becomes more severe. If the bleeding is severe, a woman will be hospitalized and blood transfusions may be necessary. If it isn't severe, complete bed rest at home is usually prescribed until the bleeding stops, then the mother will be advised to limit her physical activity. The degree of placenta previa may change during pregnancy. As the uterus enlarges, the placenta may move upward and away from the cervix. If the placenta "migrates" to a normal position, vaginal delivery is often possible. A cesarean section, however, is always done when the cervix is either totally or partially covered.

Abruptio Placenta

This is a condition in which the placenta separates from the uterine wall. The degree of separation can range from slight to complete. If only a tiny part becomes separated, it is possible that the condition will not worsen. But any separation, no matter how slight, poses a potentially serious problem. Bleeding and abdominal pain are signs of abruptio placenta. If a woman experiences any bleeding or pain, she should call her caregiver promptly. Abruptio placenta can cause maternal hemorrhage and shock and can be fatal for both the mother and the baby. If a severe separation is diagnosed, preparations will be made to deliver the baby, either vaginally or by cesarean section, depending on the individual case. In the event of a complete separation, an immediate cesarean is always done.

Premature Rupture of the Membranes (PROM)

Normally, the amniotic sac, or bag of waters, ruptures during labor. In about 10 percent of pregnancies, however, the sac ruptures before the onset of labor. If a woman is close to term, labor usually begins within 24 hours after the membranes rupture. If labor does not begin or if the pregnancy has not reached term, two potential risks arise: infection and delivery of a premature baby.

Physicians differ in how they manage PROM. If labor does not begin in a certain amount of time, some physicians induce labor if the baby is thought to be at least 33 weeks old or weighs at least 4½ pounds. The baby's weight can be estimated by doing an ultrasound scan. Other physicians, however, do not induce labor after a set period of time, but take a more conservative, wait-and-see approach. They believe that it is best to give the baby as much time as is safely possible to continue to mature. The mother is carefully monitored, and the risk of infection is continuously weighed against the risk of prematurity. If an infection is suspected, the baby is promptly delivered, either by cesarean section or by inducing labor, depending on the individual case. Some physicians routinely hospitalize women with ruptured membranes; others allow women to remain at home, with instructions to stay in bed to take their temperatures at least twice daily, and to promptly report any elevated temperature. An elevated temperature can indicate the presence of infection, as can a foul-smelling vaginal discharge.

A mother who suspects that her membranes have ruptured should call her caregiver immediately. There may be a gush of fluid or a leak. The first thing the caregiver will do is determine whether the membranes have indeed ruptured. It's not uncommon in late pregnancy for a woman to leak urine because of the enlarging uterus pressing against the bladder. Increased vaginal secretions are also common in late pregnancy. The presence of amniotic fluid is easily determined with a piece of yellow nitrazine paper. Amniotic fluid is highly alkaline and will turn the yellow paper blue.

Premature Labor

Between 7 and 10 percent of babies are born prematurely—that is, they are born at least three weeks earlier than their expected due dates. Exactly what triggers premature labor is still not known. Certain problems, however, may increase the risk of giving birth prematurely.

Women who are anemic or malnourished, for example, are at greater risk, as are women who have a previous history of premature birth or repeated miscarriage. Women who experience placental problems, toxemia, or high blood pressure during pregnancy are also at increased risk. Premature labor is more common in multiple pregnancies, too, and among women who have incompetent cervixes. In about half the cases of premature birth, however, no risk factor can be identified.

A woman who thinks she is having premature labor contractions should call her caregiver at once. If premature labor is diagnosed, the physician may try to arrest it. In certain situations, however, the safest course may be to allow labor to continue—if the mother is seriously ill, for example, or if the baby is at risk in his uterine home.

Until quite recently, the most widely used method for inhibiting premature labor was to administer alcohol intravenously. Today, however, a drug called ritodrine is most commonly used. This drug, which was approved for use by the FDA in 1980, relaxes the uterine muscles and slows down labor contractions. Ritodrine is not appropriate for all cases of premature labor, nor is it appropriate for all women. The decision to use ritodrine must be carefully made, and when it is used, the mother will be closely monitored. Under ideal conditions, ritodrine has successfully delayed the onset of labor for days and even weeks.

When premature labor cannot be arrested, the best place for the mother to be is a large medical center with a neonatal intensive care unit or preparations should be made for transferring the baby to such a facility. In the last decade, great strides have been made in saving even the smallest of babies. In most sophisticated neonatal units in this country, babies weighing between 2 and 3 pounds now have an 80 to 85 percent chance of surviving. Ten years ago, most of the 2-pounders did not make it.

Postmature Syndrome

A pregnancy is said to last 40 weeks from the first day of the last menstrual period. Most babies arrive within two weeks before or after the 40 weeks. A pregnancy that goes beyond 42 weeks is considered post-term. In a post-term pregnancy, there is the potential risk of what is called the postmature syndrome. This means that the aging placenta is degenerating and no longer supplying the baby with sufficient oxygen and nutrients. This, in turn, poses a serious threat to the baby's well-being. There are a number of tests that can be done to determine if the baby is being compromised, including estriol, nonstress, and stress tests, which are explained in the next section. If the baby is in danger, labor will be induced or a cesarean will be done, depending on the individual case. The postmature syndrome is found in about 20 percent of pregnancies that go beyond 42 weeks.

Nonroutine Tests

The routine tests that are done at the first and subsequent prenatal visits usually give a reasonably accurate picture of how a pregnancy is progressing. Occasionally, however, additional diagnostic information may be needed, especially when a complication is suspected or when a woman begins pregnancy at risk. Most expectant mothers will not be involved with the nonroutine tests discussed below, but it's helpful to know what they are and why and how they're done in case one ever becomes necessary.

Ultrasound

With this procedure, high-frequency sound waves are beamed into the body. The sound waves bounce off internal tissues and produce echoes. The echoes, in turn, are transformed into a visible image that is displayed on a screen similar to that in a television set. Ultrasound has become a valuable diagnostic tool during pregnancy because it can provide important information about what is happening inside the uterus. It can help diagnose problems with the placenta, certain fetal abnormalities, and multiple pregnancies. It can help determine fetal age and whether or not the fetus is growing at a normal rate. These determinations are made by measuring the size of the baby's skull and comparing it to standards of fetal growth.

If you go for an ultrasound scan, you will probably be asked to drink about 2 quarts of water. You will have to hold the water until the procedure is over, but this is the only discomfort associated with ultrasound. Your abdomen will be oiled, and a transducer will be gently moved over it. The transducer both directs the sound waves and picks up the echoes, which will become the picture that you will be able to see on a small TV-like screen. If real-time ultrasound is used, you will see a moving picture. If a static scanning device is used, the picture will be still. In either case, you shouldn't expect to see a clear image. The technician will probably have to interpret much of the picture for you.

To date, ultrasound is believed to be safe. Because it is a relatively new procedure, however, it is still too soon to know whether or not it has any long-term ill effects. Preliminary studies are reassuring, and other studies are currently being conducted. When medically indicated, ultrasound can provide valuable diagnostic information, but until the final verdict is in on its safety, it should not be done for curiosity's sake.

Amniocentesis

With this procedure, a thin, hollow needle is inserted through the abdomen and into the uterus, and a small amount of amniotic fluid is withdrawn for testing. Amniocentesis is most commonly used to test for genetic defects, both chromosomal abnormalities and metabolic disorders. Many of these defects are extremely rare, but some, such as Down's syndrome, are more common. Not all genetic defects, however, can be detected by amniocentesis. When used for genetic testing, amniocentesis is done between 16 and 20 weeks after the first day of the last menstrual period. Physicians wait for at least 16 weeks because they want to be sure that there is enough amniotic fluid so that the procedure can be safely done. The fluid contains cells shed by the fetus. These cells are cultured and grown in the laboratory, then they are examined for chromosomal abnormalities. In the case of metabolic disorders, the fluid undergoes biochemical analysis. It usually takes three or four weeks before the results are known. This waiting period can be an extremely anxious time for the parents. But in about 95 percent of the cases, the results are reassuring. Amniocentesis does reveal the sex of the baby. If a sex-linked disorder were suspected, the parents would, of course, be told the baby's sex. Otherwise, parents can choose either to be informed or to wait until delivery.

Amniocentesis is generally advised in the following situations: if the parents have a previous child with a defect that can be diagnosed with amniocentesis; if one or both parents are known or suspected to carry the trait for a diagnosable defect; if the mother is older than 35; and if the father is older than 55, regardless of what age the mother is. Some geneticists also believe that amniocentesis is advisable for a woman who has a previous history of three or more miscarriages.

Amniocentesis is generally recommended for women over 35 because of the increased risk of having a child with a chromosomal abnormality, especially Down's syndrome. At age 20, the risk of having a Down's syndrome baby is about 1 in 2,000; at age 35, it's about 1 in 400; at age 40, it's 1 in 105; and at age 44, it's 1 in 35. There is also a higher incidence of chromosomal abnormalities among babies whose fathers are over the age of 55.

The decision on whether or not to have amniocentesis is the parents'. Some parents decide against the procedure because of religious or ethical considerations. Parents who would not consider terminating a pregnancy may feel that the test is unnecessary, unless they simply want to be prepared. Whenever a need for amniocentesis is indicated, the parents should be carefully counseled as to the procedure and the risks and benefits that are involved. While complications are extremely rare, they do occur and include miscarriage, bleeding, and leakage of amniotic fluid. The risk of complications developing is estimated to be between ½ and 1 percent.

While it is used mainly to detect genetic defects, amniocentesis is used in other ways to evaluate the well-being of the baby. In cases of Rh disease, for example, analysis of the amniotic fluid can help determine if the baby's blood cells are being adversely affected. Analysis of the fluid can also help determine the maturity of the baby's lungs. This is often done before a scheduled cesarean section or when an early delivery is being considered because the baby is at risk in his uterine home. The lungs are the last organs to develop fully, and if the baby is born before they are sufficiently mature, there is the danger of respiratory distress syndrome.

If you have amniocentesis, an ultrasound scan will be done first to locate the position of the baby and the placenta so that neither will be punctured by the needle. Before the needle is inserted, you may be given a local anesthetic to numb the area. A growing number of physicians, however, are omitting this because the needle for amniocentesis is no more painful than the anesthetic needle. Most women say there is minimal discomfort associated with amniocentesis. Instead of pain, they usually feel a stinging sensation when the needle is inserted.

Alpha-fetoprotein (AFP) Testing

The presence of elevated levels of AFP, a protein produced by the baby, in the mother's bloodstream or in the amniotic fluid can indicate a neural tube defect, such as spina bifida or anencephaly. Spina bifida is a malformation of the baby's spinal column; anencephaly is a deformity of the skull and brain. A blood test for alpha-fetoprotein is done at about the 16th week of pregnancy. If the test is positive, another blood test is done. If the second blood test still shows abnormally high levels of AFP, the next step is an ultrasound scan. The scan can help rule out other possible causes of high AFP levels, such as a multiple pregnancy or a baby who is older than originally calculated. The scan can also determine whether or not there is a visible defect. If no defect is apparent and there is only one baby of the expected age, the next step is amniocentesis. If abnormally high levels of AFP are found in the amniotic fluid, the chance is high that a neural tube defect is present.

Estriol Testing

Estriol is a hormone formed in the placenta from other hormones that are mostly produced by the baby. Estriol enters the mother's bloodstream and is excreted in the urine, and either blood or urine samples may be used for testing. Toward the end of pregnancy, estriol testing is

Your Pregnant Body

often done in certain high-risk situations—if the mother is diabetic, for example, or if there is the possibility of postmaturity. The testing helps monitor placental function and fetal well-being. A steady or increasing level of estriol is normal; a low or falling level may mean the baby is in distress. Estriol testing is generally used before or in conjunction with nonstress and stress tests.

Nonstress Test

This procedure is done to help determine how a baby will respond to the stress of labor. In certain high-risk situations, it may be done regularly at the end of pregnancy as a means of monitoring fetal well-being. In a nonstress test, the baby's heart rate is measured with an electronic monitor, usually in the doctor's office. When the baby moves, his heart rate should accelerate by at least 15 beats per minute. If the heart rate does not increase in response to movement, the baby may be in jeopardy, and a stress test will probably be ordered.

Stress Test

This is also called the oxytocin challenge test. Oxytocin is the hormone that stimulates labor contractions, and a stress test measures the response of the fetal heart to contractions. For this procedure, the mother must be in the hospital. She is given just enough oxytocin intravenously to induce three good contractions, and the baby's heart rate is monitored electronically. A decrease in the heart rate is a danger signal, which usually calls for prompt delivery of the baby.

The nonroutine tests make it possible to discover potential problems. But there is something that you can do on your own to help monitor your baby's health. Recent research has demonstrated that movement is one of the best indications of the unborn baby's well-being. Each baby shows a different pattern of movement, and you'll become familiar with your baby's pattern during the months of pregnancy. All babies have active periods and rest periods; you should not be alarmed if you haven't felt your baby move for an hour or so. But it's important to report a sudden change in the pattern or in the amount of movement. A general guideline is that if your baby makes less than three movements in a 12-hour period, you should call your caregiver.

3. Your Pregnant Self

Pregnancy is a transitional state of being. It is neither childlessness nor parenthood, but in a sense it is both. During these nine months, a new human being is developing and getting ready for independent life. At the same time, her parents must prepare themselves for their new roles and for the arrival of the new person who will be changing their lives. No wonder pregnancy is such an emotional time for most women and men. From the moment of conception, you have embarked on a journey with only a very sketchy map. But the journey is as exciting as it is scary, and its length, at least, is pretty much a certainty.

Emotional Ups and Downs

Pregnancy is often described as an emotional roller coaster, with highs and lows and a lot of mixed feelings. Emotional changeability is entirely appropriate given the circumstances. Whether this baby was planned or not, whether he is your first or your fourth, he will undoubtedly change your life just as he is now changing your physical appearance. No matter how much a baby is wanted, nearly every expectant parent thinks at some point that he or she has made a mistake and should not be having a child. Almost everyone experiences at least some ambivalence, fear, and resentment, together with happy feelings of anticipation and fulfillment. These conflicting emotions are a normal part of pregnancy.

In many respects, pregnancy is a rehearsal for parenthood, as you and your husband evaluate the type of parents you will be and how your lives will be different once your baby arrives. Both of you will have many concerns and questions during these nine months, and it's essential that they be discussed and put into perspective. While there's little doubt that pregnancy constitutes an emotional crisis for a woman and a man, it is equally true that it offers rich opportunities for growth and fulfillment, both as individuals and as a couple. These nine months can be as rewarding as they can be trying, and for many couples, they are a time of new understanding and intimacy.

While each woman and man will respond to pregnancy in a unique way, there are concerns that are common to most pregnancies. Researchers have also found that expectant parents often have similar concerns during each of the three trimesters.

Your Pregnant Self

The First Trimester

During the first few months, a woman is usually struggling to accept the reality of the pregnancy. Even if it is planned and fervently wanted, actually having the pregnancy confirmed may bring forth an ambivalence that may surprise and confuse you. The physical discomforts of the first trimester verify that you are pregnant, yet can make you miserable and question why you became pregnant. You may worry that you are imagining that you are pregnant and that the laboratory made a mistake. Such fears are indications of ambivalence. On the one hand, you want the pregnancy so much that you're afraid you're just imagining it. But on the other hand, you secretly hope that it's all in your head, because you're not sure you'll be able to cope. Ambivalent feelings are not only normal, they're very useful, as they help a woman accept the reality of the pregnancy. You may also find that you are anxious for the baby to move and for the pregnancy to show so that expecting a baby won't be such an abstract concept.

Extreme mood swings are common during the first trimester. A woman may find herself elated one moment and, for no apparent reason, depressed the next. Emotional reactions to unrelated things are also common. Says one new mother, "I remember becoming hysterical because my husband didn't take out the garbage." Another woman, pregnant with her second child, says, "I knew I was pregnant even before the test confirmed it, when I started crying over commercials for toothpaste." Some women become emotional looking at pictures of babies or even walking through the layette department of a store. Increased hormonal levels no doubt play a part in these heightened emotions and mood swings. Especially in the early months, when a woman's body is adjusting to this rapid increase, certain hormones can intensify feelings that are already present.

During the first trimester, you may also find yourself staring at mothers, babies, and other pregnant women, even though you may never have given them a second glance before. It's almost as if the mothers have a secret and you can discern the answer just by looking.

A man may be more emotionally distant from the pregnancy during the early months. His body is not undergoing radical change, nor is the pregnancy visible. Yet while he may have difficulty relating to the pregnancy, he can't help but wonder what impact the baby will have on his life. Some men also experience physical symptoms that parallel those of their pregnant wives, such as nausea, fatigue, and backache. This physical identification with the expectant mother is known as the couvade syndrome, from the French word *couver*, meaning "to brood" or "to hatch." It most commonly occurs during the first few months of pregnancy and may reoccur as birth becomes imminent. Informal observations suggest that perhaps 50 percent of expectant fathers experience pregnancy-related symptoms.

The Second Trimester

Two things happen during this trimester that help make the pregnancy and baby more of a reality: the pregnancy begins to show and the first fetal movements can be felt, usually at about four and a half months. The first time she feels her baby move is a powerful and significant moment for a woman. Finally, there is physical confirmation of the baby's existence. At the same time, she begins to perceive the baby as a separate individual. The baby's first movements are usually too delicate for the father to detect; in a few weeks, however, the baby will become large and active enough so that the father can see and feel the movements when he puts his hand on his wife's abdomen. From this point, most expectant parents find that they feel closer to the baby. They begin to think about names, about whom the baby will look like, and about what it will be like to have a baby. You may also find yourself turning inward and listening more to your internal self, at once communing with the baby inside you and feeling far away from the external world.

As you begin to perceive the baby as a separate individual, you may also begin to worry about whether she is healthy and normal. Her movements reassure you that she is alive, but they can't reassure you that she is perfect. Many expectant fathers also have anxieties about the baby's health and normalcy, and it's essential that both parents get such concerns out into the open, where they can be discussed and put into perspective.

You may have a variety of reactions when your pregnancy begins to show. You will probably feel very happy and proud, but you may also feel a bit dismayed about your changing contours. Many women worry about how their bodies will react to pregnancy. Some women are distressed by the changes that take place; other women revel in them. How you feel about being pregnant can affect how you feel about your changing body. And your changing body can affect how you feel about being pregnant. Most women vacillate between feeling attractive and feeling unattractive throughout their pregnancies. Having a supportive husband can be a great comfort when you're feeling unbeguiling. "My husband was always quick to say how beautiful I looked," says one new mother. "He helped ease my fears that he would lose interest in me, and he helped me appreciate my pregnant body." Men also have varied reactions to their wives' changing contours. Some men are delighted and find their pregnant wives especially desirable; other men are disturbed by the changes, which could indicate that they haven't yet come to terms with the pregnancy or the fact that they will soon be fathers.

During the second trimester, you may find yourself thinking a lot about your own mother and your relationship with her, especially during your childhood years. In examining the way you were raised, you are helping to forge your own identity as a parent. You may begin to see your mother in a more compassionate and accepting light, now that you are about to become a mother yourself. Many women forgive their mothers for not being everything they wanted them to be. "I was so preoccupied with whether I'd be a good mother, and I was terrified that I'd be like mine," says one expectant mother. "But the pregnancy has made me want to resolve everything with her, and I've begun to think that maybe she did the best she could." Understanding your mother and forgiving her for any mistakes and shortcomings can help you come to terms with your own fallibility. "I'm forgiving everyone I can get my hands on," says another expectant mother. "Maybe then I'll be able to forgive myself for the mistakes I know I'm going to make." Older women who are pregnant for the first time may not have to resolve as many issues with their mothers. "It's true that I thought a lot about my mother and that I had a lot of questions," says one new mother in her late thirties. "But the pregnancy didn't bring me a new relationship with her. That had already happened."

Expectant fathers usually go through a similar period of examining how they were raised and what type of parents their fathers were. It may be more difficult for an expectant father to consider his own father as a role model, since the father's role has changed considerably in recent years. His own father may have been very traditional—the sole breadwinner and the "heavy" in the family who held tight rein on his emotions. Still, an expectant father will probably begin to see his father in a new and more accepting light.

As you and your husband examine your relationships with your parents, you may also begin to examine your relationship with each other. Pregnancy may make you feel more bound to each other and your relationship may seem more permanent than ever before. Because of this, you may for a time be more critical of each other. You may also find that you are giving serious thought to what type of parent the other will be.

Another concern that often arises during the second trimester is the issue of dependency. Being pregnant may make you feel dependent on your husband in a way you never did before, and this may make you anxious and uncomfortable. You may also realize that having a child will certainly make you even more dependent on him. Your husband, on the other hand, may be grappling with the reality that two people will be dependent on him. Coming to terms with the dependency issue is part of the mental work of pregnancy.

The Third Trimester

By the last trimester, the baby is clearly perceived as a separate individual, and the pregnancy is an inescapable reality. Many concerns will have been put into perspective, and you will find yourself thinking more and more about the impending birth. What will labor be like? How painful will it be? Will you get through it well? Will your husband be supportive? Anxieties about birth are not only natural but also serve a very useful purpose, as they help prepare you for the emotional and physical work of labor and delivery. Studies show that women who are conscious of their fears about birth, and who are able to express and discuss them, often find labor less difficult than women who keep their anxieties suppressed or unexpressed. Your husband will likely be having his own worries about the birth, and they probably serve a similar purpose as your concerns. Will he be a good labor coach? How will he feel watching the birth? Will you get through labor okay? Many husbands also have irrational fears about their wives'

Your Pregnant Self

well-being. "During the last few weeks, I was preoccupied with the thought that something terrible was going to happen to my wife during birth," says one new father. "I knew I was being irrational. Still, I didn't calm down until the baby was actually born and I could see that my wife was absolutely fine." As the birth draws closer, you and your husband may also feel that everything is getting out of control. The baby is growing, labor will begin, and the baby will be born whether or not you want him to—and nature will choose when and how, not you.

During the last trimester, as the abdomen grows larger, the pregnant body becomes increasingly burdensome. You may find yourself more fatigued and uncomfortable than at any other time during your pregnancy. By the eighth or ninth month, you may begin to feel that you have been pregnant forever, and you may be anxious to get it all over with. At the same time, however, you may be a bit sad that the pregnancy is coming to an end.

Thoughts about the baby and what it will be like to have a baby become more persistent as the birth day approaches. You may also find yourself wondering whether there will be enough love for everyone once the baby does arrive. This is a common concern of both expectant mothers and fathers, and like all the other questions and concerns of pregnancy, it should be examined and discussed.

There is a special need for good communication during these nine months, when feelings of happiness and fulfillment are all mixed up with doubts and worries. If you and your husband keep in mind that certain concerns are a natural part of pregnancy and that they serve a useful purpose, it should be easier for each of you to express them when they arise. You will both probably be very surprised at how similar many of your feelings are. The emotional challenges of pregnancy are great, but the rewards are too. These nine months offer us a unique opportunity to gain new insights into ourselves and our spouses, and in the end to be more responsive parents.

Pregnancy Dreams

Dreams during pregnancy are usually quite vivid, and expectant parents often find that they think a lot about their dreams. Pregnancy dreams can be pleasant, even euphoric, or they can be bizarre and frightening.

Expectant fathers as well as mothers have dreams about giving birth, either to a real baby or to some type of animal or creature. After the birth, the parent may lose the baby or put it someplace, such as in a closet or on a shelf. Both men and women also have dreams about taking care of a baby, who is usually at least several months old and quite pretty and charming. Dreams about deformed babies are also common among men and women. Expectant mothers, however, are much more likely to have dreams where they identify with the fetus. In early pregnancy, for example, a woman may dream that she is floating or swimming in a pool of water. As the birth draws near, she may dream about falling through a narrow opening or space.

A dream, of course, can only be interpreted by the person who had the dream. In addition, dreams can be interpreted on many different levels. Say, for example, that a woman dreams about being trapped in a tight place.

She may be identifying with her baby, or the dream may signify that she has unconscious concerns that she is trapped in pregnancy or that she will be trapped in motherhood. A dream about losing the baby may mean that the parent has unresolved questions about how the baby will change his life or that he hasn't yet come to terms with the fact that he will soon be a father. Dreams about older babies might signify any number of things: a parent's inexperience with a newborn, a refusal to think about how helpless a newborn is, or simply a pleasant reverie about what life will be like with a baby. Then again, it might be a wish-fulfillment dream. After all, wouldn't it be nice to have a lovely baby without having to go through childbirth?

Unfortunately, expectant parents tend to view pleasant dreams as good signs and frightening dreams as ominous signs. In reality, however, dreams cannot possibly predict either what type of parent you will be or what your baby will be like. Dreams about deformed babies, for example, simply signify a parent's natural concern about her baby's health and normalcy. Dreams can, however, serve the very useful function of helping you resolve some of your anxieties about the baby and about the birth, about what type of parent you will be, and about how the baby will change your life. Often, a dream can alert you to some anxiety or attitude before you are even consciously aware of it.

Dr. Robert Gillman, a Washington psychiatrist, studied the dreams of 44 first-time expectant mothers and rated the dreams according to the presence of masochistic and hostile elements. The women were then studied after their babies were born and rated according to how well they adapted to their roles as mothers. Dr. Gillman compared the dream ratings with the adaptation ratings and found that the dreams did not predict how well the women would adapt to their new roles.

Another study of the relationship between pregnant women's dreams and the length of labor is particularly reassuring. The researchers found that the more anxious a woman's dreams were, the shorter her labor was. Having worked out many of their anxieties in their dreams, the women were apparently better able to relax during labor.

If you or your husband has a frightening dream, share it with each other. Once it's out in the open, you can begin to look at it objectively. At the very least, you'll feel relieved when the dream is verbalized and discussed. It might also act as a springboard for discussing some fear or worry that you and your spouse have not talked about before. Be sure to share your pleasant dreams too. Feeling good and looking forward together can bring a heightened sense of intimacy and fulfillment.

You may have thought that only your body would undergo a metamorphosis during pregnancy, but as you can see, your feelings and your husband's feelings also change dramatically. Bodily changes nurture your baby and prepare him for life outside the womb; emotional changes prepare you and your husband for your new roles as parents.

Sex and the Expectant Couple

Sex—it's what got this baby business started in the first place. Yet now that you are pregnant, you and your husband may have questions and concerns about your sexual relationship. Until quite recently, sex during pregnancy was a subject that was rarely discussed or studied. This may help explain why many expectant parents are unprepared for the impact that the physical and emotional changes of pregnancy can have on their feelings of sexuality. In addition, misconceptions about sex during pregnancy linger on and can contribute to some couples' feelings of uncertainty about sex.

One fear that persists is that sexual intercourse can somehow harm the baby. When pregnancy is progressing normally, this fear is groundless. The baby is well insulated, enclosed within the amniotic sac inside the uterus, and the cervix is sealed with the mucous plug. Another common worry is that intercourse during the first trimester can cause a miscarriage. Again, in a normal pregnancy, this concern is unfounded. A woman who has a previous history of miscarriage, however, is usually advised to abstain from intercourse during early pregnancy. The chief consideration is not penetration, but orgasm. Although the findings are inconclusive, some researchers feel that orgasm and the uterine contractions that normally follow could lead to miscarriage in women who are already at risk.

Certain conditions may arise during pregnancy that would call for sexual abstinence, including spotting or bleeding, placenta previa, and threatened premature labor. But in a pregnancy where no complicating factors arise, a couple can continue to enjoy sexual relations. The subject of sex should be discussed with your physician or nurse-midwife, who can advise you according to the individual circumstances of your pregnancy. Many expectant parents feel uncomfortable or embarrassed approaching their caregivers with questions about sex, and it is only fair to point out that many caregivers are also uncomfortable discussing the subject. Even so, they are usually prepared to answer questions, especially those concerning safety. It may be up to you, however, to initiate the discussion, and you shouldn't feel timid. Sexual loving is too important a part of a couple's relationship to let unfounded worries get in the way. At the same time, you should be aware of how the physical and emotional changes of pregnancy can influence the sexual relationship.

The First Trimester

The physical discomforts of early pregnancy often leave a woman with a diminished interest in sex. Her husband may respond to this with understanding or annoyance, or he may be of two minds. He may see his wife's lack of desire as a rejection of him, rather than simply a natural response to being physically uncomfortable. Emotional factors can also play a part in decreased sexual interest. A woman may be preoccupied with trying to accept the reality of the pregnancy. She may be experiencing mood swings, intensified by increased hormonal levels. Or she

Your Pregnant Self

may be unconsciously worried about miscarriage and that can put a damper on sexual interest too.

For some women, however, the first trimester is a time of increased sexual desire. If a woman is not experiencing much discomfort from nausea or fatigue, these months can be a continuation of the preconception period, when sex was probably very pleasurable because birth control was unnecessary. In fact, the knowledge that conception has occurred can bring an enjoyable spontaneity to a couple's sex life because they have been released from the pressure of trying to conceive. And the knowledge that they have created a new life together often increases the pleasure that a woman and a man find in each other.

In addition to such common discomforts as nausea and fatigue, there are other physical changes that can influence sexual relations. The breasts, for example, begin to enlarge very early in pregnancy, and they and the nipples are usually very tender and sensitive to touch. There may be discomfort or even pain when the breasts and nipples are caressed. This tenderness passes, but in the meantime, a couple may have to adjust their sex play to avoid breast discomfort. Many men find their wives' enlarged breasts particularly erotic.

An increase in vaginal discharge is typical during pregnancy and usually begins during the first trimester. The increased discharge means that you are more lubricated, making penetration easier. However, it generally brings a change in the smell and taste of the vaginal area, which may not be arousing to your husband if oral sex is a normal part of your lovemaking. Showering just before making love or using scented oils can help if this is a problem for you. You should not douche during pregnancy.

There is one manifestation of sex play that definitely should *not* be practiced during pregnancy: blowing air into the vagina. This is dangerous at any time but is especially so during pregnancy, because the veins of the vagina and cervix are enlarged and dilated. Air can enter the mother's bloodstream via the veins and cause an air embolism, which can be fatal to the mother.

The Second Trimester

For many women, the middle months of pregnancy are a time of increased sexual desire. A number of factors may contribute to this heightened sexuality. The physical discomforts of early pregnancy are generally gone, and a woman may experience a new sense of vitality and well-being. While the pregnancy begins to show, the abdomen is not yet so large as to be obtrusive. Any conscious or unconscious fears of miscarriage will have vanished, and emotionally, the woman may have come to terms with the reality of the pregnancy. In addition, physical changes in the pelvic area can heighten sexual sensitivity and increase a woman's capacity for orgasm. During sexual arousal, blood naturally flows to the pelvic area. Following orgasm, the blood slowly flows away from the area. During pregnancy, the pelvic area is naturally congested with blood, and this can heighten sexual sensitivity. One woman describes the way she felt during the second trimester as being "always ready." Researchers have found that some women experience their first orgasm during this period; others experience multiple orgasms for the first time. Following orgasm, an expectant mother may ex-

Your Pregnant Self

perience an unusually prolonged period of sexual tension, because it takes longer for the blood to leave the pelvic area than it does when she isn't pregnant.

How a woman feels about her changing contours and how her husband feels about them will, of course, have an influence on the sexual relationship. The perception of fetal movement, which usually occurs during the middle of this trimester, can also have an effect on sexual feelings. Some couples incorporate these new feelings of life into their lovemaking. The movements are simply another form of touching and one more thing about the body to be noticed and enjoyed. Other couples simply ignore them. Some men and women, however, are disturbed by the movements. Some feel that the baby is somehow aware of what is happening, and even though they may realize that this can't possibly be so, they just can't seem to shake the notion that a third party is present. Other men and women find that the movements distract them from lovemaking and get them thinking about other things. The movements are, after all, clear evidence of the baby's existence and a reminder of impending parenthood.

The Third Trimester

As the abdomen gets larger, the male superior, or man-on-top, position will be uncomfortable. If this is the position that you and your husband usually assume for intercourse, you will have to try new positions. Many couples find that the female superior, or woman-on-top, position or the side-by-side position is the most comfortable and enjoyable for both the woman and the man.

Many women find that sexual desire decreases during the last trimester. Physical factors no doubt play a part in diminished desire. The body becomes particularly burdensome as pregnancy progresses, and you will probably feel very fatigued and uncomfortable. Your husband may also be less interested in sex. In fact, the two of you may have similar reasons for a lack of interest. Some women find it difficult to feel sexy when their bodies are so different from the ones they and society tend to perceive as sexually appealing. "At the end, you get so big that it's hard to envision yourself as a love goddess," quips one women in her ninth month. And even men who find the pregnant body very erotic may be a bit overwhelmed by the size of the abdomen at eight or nine months. You and your husband may also be preoccupied with mental preparations for childbirth and final preparations for the baby and parenthood—both physical and mental. And the fact that intercourse becomes increasingly cumbersome can add to the disinterest. ("All the books tell you to be creative in sex. Give me a break!" laughs another woman late in her pregnancy.) Sex may also not be as fulfilling for a woman during the final months. By the last trimester, the pelvic area is so congested or engorged with blood that a woman may have difficulty reaching orgasm, even though she may be very aroused. This can be frustrating. Even when orgasm or multiple orgasms are attained, they may not relieve sexual tension because there is so much blood in the area. This too, can be frustrating.

For some couples, however, the third trimester does not bring a decline in sexual desire. In fact, some see it as a last chance for spontaneous lovemaking. "It's sort of a time bomb theory," explains one expectant mother.

"Nearing the end, you think you have to do it on the chandeliers, because you'll never do it again. You're afraid you'll change and never have sex again once the baby is born." But even this woman found that sex wasn't quite as satisfying during the final months as it had been earlier. "I've had a lot better. I wouldn't want to do this all the time," she says. "Half of me wants wild weekends and the other half doesn't want to be bothered."

Until quite recently, doctors routinely advised against sexual relations during the last weeks of pregnancy. While this prohibition is not as routine as it once was, many physicians still adhere to it. Whether or not intercourse during the last month or so poses a risk in a normal pregnancy has been the focus of much attention in recent years. Relatively few studies have been conducted and the results are often contradictory. Some researchers believe that the uterine contractions that follow orgasm are strong enough to possibly initiate labor near the end of pregnancy. Other researchers, however, have found no correlation between orgasm and a higher incidence of premature labor in uncomplicated pregnancies. Another reason for advising abstinence in late pregnancy is to guard against the possibility of infection, and here, too, research findings are contradictory. Some studies have found a higher incidence of infection among babies born to women who had intercourse during the last month of pregnancy than among women who didn't. But other studies have found no difference in infection rates between women who abstained and women who did not. Intercourse is definitely contraindicated once the bag of waters has ruptured, as bacteria can invade the uterus when the membranes are no longer intact. And, of course, if a woman is at risk—if she has a history of premature labor, for example, or is experiencing symptoms of premature labor, or if there is spotting or bleeding—abstinence would be called for.

Whether your caregiver advises abstinence at the end of pregnancy or whether she believes that sexual relations can be continued, you should discuss the reasons with her. In the end, each couple must reach their own decision, and it should be one that is based on facts and understanding.

Each Experience Is Unique

Research on sex during pregnancy has shown that there is no set pattern to how expectant parents respond sexually. Some couples experience a decline of interest in the first trimester, an upsurge in the second, then a decline in the third. Others experience a steady decline over the nine-month period, while some couples experience a steady increase. And even within the different patterns, there are wide variations from day to day or week to week.

What's most important is that you and your husband share your feelings about sex. Understanding between a husband and wife and sensitivity to each other's sexual needs are important at any time, but especially during pregnancy when so many physical and emotional factors can influence feelings of sexuality.

4. Lifestyle

Not too long ago, pregnancy meant retirement for women—retirement from leisure activities as well as from work. Attitudes, however, have changed since your mother was expecting you, and pregnancy is no longer seen as an illness or an embarrassment. Your lifestyle need not be altered drastically just because you are expecting. If your pregnancy is progressing normally, you can continue to enjoy most activities that you are already accustomed to—albeit with some moderation and minor adjustments. Keeping active during these nine months can help you feel good about yourself and can help make the time go faster too.

On the Job

Whatever type of work you may do, you will probably have many questions about working while you are pregnant. When and how should you tell your employer? Will your pregnancy change your relationship with your boss and your co-workers? Will pregnancy have any effect on your work? Will any modifications have to be made in the work that you do? Are you entitled to any benefits? Do you have any legal rights?

The answer to the last question is simple—yes you do! The Pregnancy Discrimination Act, which was signed into law in 1978 as an amendment to Title VII of the 1964 Civil Rights Act, is your guarantee that you cannot be legally discriminated against because of pregnancy, childbirth, or *related medical conditions*. This amendment means that you are not only protected against discrimination in such areas as firing, promotions, and mandatory leaves, but that you are also entitled to any health, disability, or sick-leave benefits that your employer may offer. In other words, pregnancy and birth cannot be treated differently from any other medical disability. If an employer provides health insurance, maternity coverage must be included. If he provides temporary payments for people who are unable to work because of medical disability, he must do the same for pregnancy and birth. It should be pointed out that the law does not require employers to start new benefit programs if they don't already exist, nor does it require them to give pregnant women preferential treatment. In addition, the law applies only to companies with 15 or more employees, although some states have passed their own laws to include smaller companies too.

Benefits

Early in pregnancy, you should find out what your company's policies are regarding disability benefits and

Lifestyle

maternity leave, and you should check out your health insurance. Most companies have written policy statements for employees, and most supply handbooks that outline insurance coverage. If you've misplaced yours or can't recall receiving one, ask in your personnel department.

Having a baby can be an expensive proposition, and your health insurance is going to be very important to you. Just because maternity coverage must be included in any health insurance plan provided by your employer, you should not assume that every medical expense is going to be covered. More than likely it will not be. To help you plan for any expenses that you may be responsible for, you should find out as soon as possible exactly what type of coverage you have. Health insurance plans vary significantly from one company to another. Read your insurance handbook, and if you need further clarification, which you probably will, speak with your personnel department or contact the carrier directly. And be sure to find out when coverage begins for the baby, as well as the extent of the coverage.

Temporary disability payments also vary from company to company. Some employers pay full salary during the disability period others pay partial salary, and some pay nothing. Other benefits, such as health insurance, are usually continued, but do check to be sure. Remember, if an employer does not provide payments for other temporary disabilities, he is not required to do so for pregnancy and birth. If your employer is one who does not, you may be eligible for unemployment or temporary disability payments from your state. Not all states, however, provide such coverage. To find out if yours does, contact your local state employment office, department of labor, or human rights commission. Temporary disability benefits are only for the period of time that you are unable to work, and your disability must be verified by your caregiver. In addition, if you do not plan to return to work, you are not eligible for disability benefits.

The issue of maternity leave can be a separate one from disability or sick leave. Whether or not your employer provides disability coverage, he may offer an unpaid leave of absence for a certain period of time, such as three or six months. In one survey of large U.S. corporations, 65 percent offered maternity leave of up to six months without pay. Even if your employer does not have an official maternity leave policy, he may be open to granting such a leave. This type of extended leave, however, is not covered by the Pregnancy Discrimination Act, which is based on your ability to work. If you can take a leave of absence in addition to disability or sick leave, be sure to find out if your health insurance coverage will continue during the time that you are on unpaid leave. Some companies continue this benefit; others do not.

Occupational Safety

During your first prenatal visit, your caregiver should discuss the type of work you do, and she should also take an occupational history. This will help her evaluate the safety of your work routine and environment. For most women, no major adjustments will have to be made in their work routines. There are, however, some types of work that should be avoided during pregnancy; these include jobs that require constant motion, delicate balance, heavy lifting, or long periods of standing, as well as jobs

Lifestyle

that expose a woman to toxic dusts and chemicals.

What effect occupational hazards may have on pregnancy and the unborn baby is a relatively new area of investigation, and there are few definitive guidelines. Certain agents are known to pose a potential risk to the baby; these include lead, mercury, vinyl chloride, carbon monoxide, benzene, ionizing radiation, and anesthetic gases, to name a few. And there are other agents that are strongly suspected. High levels of physical stress and noise may also be harmful to the fetus.

If your work involves exposure to any toxic substance, be sure to discuss it with your caregiver. If you are uncertain about the toxicity of any substance, contact the National Institute for Occupational Safety and Health (NIOSH). For the nearest NIOSH office, look under "U.S. Government, Health and Human Services Department" in your telephone directory. If there isn't a listing, call the NIOSH office in Cincinnati, Ohio. The number is 513-684-8328.

If a major adjustment must be made in your work routine, do you have any legal protection? According to the Pregnancy Discrimination Act, an employer must treat an expectant mother who is temporarily unable to perform the functions of her job because of her pregnancy-related condition in the same manner that he treats other employees who are temporarily disabled. If, for example, he provides modified tasks or alternative assignments for other partially disabled employees, he must do the same for pregnant women. If an expectant mother believes she is being discriminated against in this or any other area of employment, she should contact her local equal employment opportunity commission or speak with her shop steward if she is a member of a union.

Telling Your Boss

Most expectant mothers have at least a few qualms about telling their employers that they are pregnant. Even if your pride and happiness are abundant, thinking about telling your boss can put a damper on your enthusiasm, because it's hard to really know how she will react.

Some women choose to inform their employers as early in pregnancy as possible. This can have certain advantages: you can stop worrying about your boss's response; you may receive some consideration from your employer or co-workers if you are feeling particularly ill during the first trimester; and you have more time to make plans with your boss either for your temporary absence or your departure from the company. Employers, in general, are grateful for as much advance notice as you are willing to give.

Other women, however, prefer to wait a few months before breaking the news. Some may be worried about miscarrying and don't want to start the ball rolling at work until the pregnancy is fairly well established. Other women, especially if the pregnancy wasn't planned, need time to sort out their feelings about the pregnancy and what they want to do career-wise. If you are worried that your employer or co-workers are going to react negatively to your pregnancy, you may want to wait as long as possible before breaking the news.

Whether you decide to tell as soon as the pregnancy test comes back positive or to wait until you begin to show will depend on many variables. But whenever you think the time is right, you should have decided on an approach, and you should be able to lay out your plans to your boss. For some employer personalities, a matter-of-fact approach—even in a memo if you can't manage it in person—is the best tack. For others, an enthusiastic announcement expressing your positive attitude, followed by a discussion of your plans, will set the right tone.

Tell your boss when you expect to deliver, how long you plan to work during pregnancy, and when you expect to return to work. Discussing your plans doesn't mean they can't be changed, but having some plans lets your boss know that you are giving serious thought to the effect that your absence will have on her and on your department. You should also discuss how your work will be done during your absence, and you should offer to train your replacement, whether you plan to return to work or not.

One magazine editor, for example, discussed taking a three-month leave of absence with her employer. She suggested that she participate in hiring a temporary replacement and that the replacement might begin work before she went on leave. The overlap would help the replacement orient herself to the job and ease the transition for everyone. When it was time to tell her boss, a pregnant social worker requested the standard six-month leave. Before she went on leave, she attached informative notes to each case file and left instructions for her replacement to call her at home if she had any questions during the leave. Whether you will be involved in the office while you are on leave depends on the type of work you do, on your particular employer, your own personality, and even on the length of your leave. A schoolteacher who was in her fourth month when school finished in June decided not to return to work in the fall, although she wasn't due to deliver until November. She and her employer felt that would be best, since she planned to take a six-month leave after the birth. She did, however, agree to substitute teach in the fall and was available to answer questions and help plan curriculum in the months before she gave birth.

Work Sense

While major job modifications will not be necessary for most expectant mothers, some minor adjustments in the work routine may be called for. Pregnancy puts extra demands on nearly every part of your body, and you are going to tire more easily. You should be sure that your job provides sufficient breaks for rest and relaxation. You should be aware, too, that fatigue can influence your job performance, especially during the first and last trimesters. You may have to curtail outside activities and go to bed much earlier at night to compensate. If you live close to work, going home for a nap at lunchtime may be a solution. If you have your own office or if there's a cot or couch in the ladies' lounge, you may be able to nap at work.

Frequent changes of position are also advisable to keep your circulation moving, and you should try to alternate sitting with standing tasks. When you do sit, keep your legs comfortably parted and your feet flat on the floor. Do not cross your legs, because this puts pressure on the veins and impedes circulation. Whenever possible, prop

Lifestyle

your feet on a footstool or other sturdy object. If your job involves a lot of standing, try not to stay in any one position for too long a time. Every once in a while, move up and down on your toes, or rock back and forth from one foot to the other. Whenever possible, sit down and elevate your legs.

Depending on where and how you get to work, commuting may or may not be a problem for you. If you work in a crowded city and depend on public transportation, it's a good idea to try to avoid peak commuter hours, especially in the later months. You might want to ask your employer for a more flexible work schedule. By coming in and leaving either a little earlier or later, you may be able to avoid rush-hour commuting. If you normally drive to work, you can usually continue doing so, as long as you fit comfortably behind the wheel. After that, you should leave the driving to someone else. Always be sure to wear your seat belt. Buckle it low, under the abdomen and across the pelvis. The shoulder harness gives added protection but should not be worn alone.

While most pregnant workers are determined that pregnancy will not make any difference in their job performance, they are often surprised that they do feel some desire to be pampered at work. These contradictory feelings often go unacknowledged but create internal conflict. You may be bent on proving that your pregnancy is beside the point and yet would appreciate some kindness and acknowledgment that you may not be feeling totally up to par. There is no solution to this predicament, but being aware of it and knowing that you are not alone in your feelings can help you to cope.

Your co-workers can also have an effect on your emotional outlook at work. They can sometimes make your life miserable, either by jealousy because they feel you're receiving preferential treatment, or by nit-picking because they think your pregnancy and leave will mean more work for them. On the other hand, co-workers can be wonderfully supportive, giving you a hand if and when you need it, and helping you sort out your feelings about work and motherhood. Even if you were sure that you wanted to return to work or that you wanted to be a full-time mother, you may find yourself having second thoughts. Nearly everyone does. Discussing the pros and cons of combining work and motherhood with women who are doing it can help you put your own thoughts into perspective.

Keeping Fit

Your mother may have been cautioned not to do any exercise during pregnancy—except housework, of course! Your own caregiver's advice, however, is more likely to be that exercise is good for you. A trip to your local bookstore will prove how attitudes have changed. You can choose from any number of books with exercise programs devised especially for pregnancy, and some suggested readings are given in the bibliography. There are also many exercise classes for expectant mothers. Especially if you're a beginner, a class has a decided advantage because an instructor is there to guide you. But whether they're experienced or not, many women find it inspiring to be exercising with other pregnant women, and they often make friends who will remain buddies post-

Lifestyle

partum. In addition to private exercise studios, many YM-YWCAs and YM-YWHAs offer special exercise programs for pregnant women, and they are usually reasonably priced.

A regular exercise program can pay triple dividends for an expectant mother. It can help ease some of the common discomforts of pregnancy; it can help prepare her body for the physical stresses of labor and delivery; and it can help speed her recovery after childbirth. Exercise is also a great way to relieve tension.

Each pregnancy, of course, is unique, and before you begin or continue any exercise program, you should consult your physician or nurse-midwife. She can best advise you because she knows your medical history and how your pregnancy is progressing. Even when you have your caregiver's okay, there are some precautions to keep in mind. One of the most important is to be sensitive to your body and stop exercising at the first sign of fatigue. If you followed a regular exercise program before pregnancy, you will probably have more stamina than if you are just beginning. All pregnant women tire more easily, however, and find it more difficult to recover from fatigue. Being sensitive to your body also means adapting your exercise routine to the changes that pregnancy brings. If an exercise feels uncomfortable or is awkward to do, discontinue it. And if an exercise ever causes pain, stop doing it. You are either doing the exercise incorrectly or have surpassed your body's limits for the moment.

Try to set aside about 20 minutes each day for exercising. A daily routine is the best way to get results. If you can exercise only a few times a week, be careful not to overdo it. Wear clothing that allows for easy movement, such as a leotard or sweat pants and a roomy T-shirt. Choose an area of your home that is carpeted and where there is enough open space so that you can exercise without having to worry about bumping into something.

Whether or not you follow a formal exercise program during pregnancy, there are a number of simple exercises that you can do to help strengthen certain muscle groups and to help you feel more comfortable. Many of these exercises can be incorporated into your daily life, at work or at home. You can do them at different times during the day, whenever you have a free moment or whenever the need strikes. Some of the following may not even seem like exercises, but nonetheless, they can be very beneficial.

Pelvic Rock

Done daily, this exercise helps relieve lower backache and abdominal pressure. It adapts well to home or work, because it can be done on hands and knees, as well as while standing or sitting. To do it, tighten your abdominal wall by pulling in and up, and tuck in your buttocks. This should straighten the natural curve in your lower back.

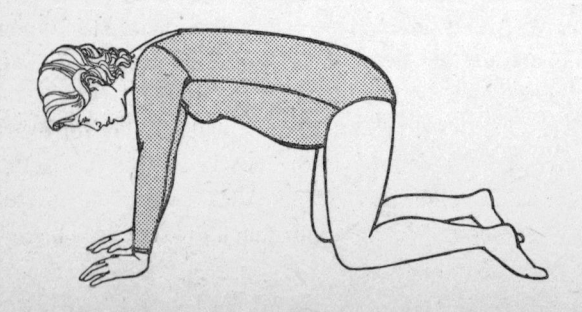

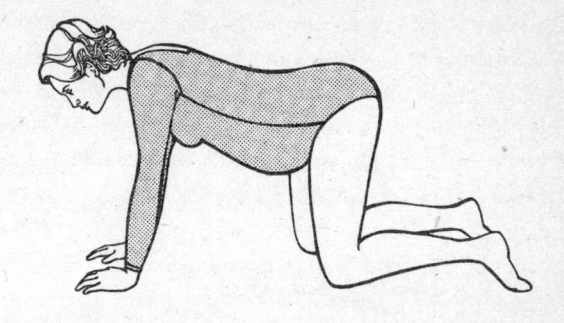

Next, slowly relax your abdomen and buttocks so that the natural curve of your back returns. Do *not* accentuate this curve. This is very important, especially in the hands and knees position. You do *not* want a hollow to form and your abdomen to sag. Pelvic rocking should be done slowly and rhythmically, and do not hold your breath when doing this or the other exercises. Continue to breathe normally. Repeat pelvic rock five or six times.

Shoulder Circling

This exercise helps relieve upper backache and can be done while standing or sitting. Let your arms hang loosely at your sides. Lift your shoulders up toward your ears, then rotate your shoulders back as far as they will comfortably go. Relax to starting position. Repeat five or six times, remembering to breathe normally.

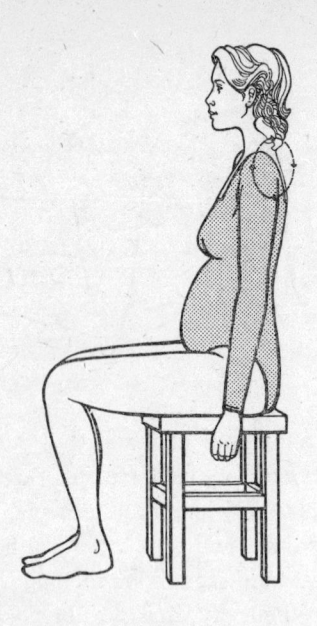

Squatting

During pregnancy, you should never bend from the waist. Whenever you must reach something at floor level, you should squat. Squatting may not seem like an exercise, but it's a good way to help strengthen muscles in the legs. You can practice squatting whenever you must get down to floor level—to open a bottom drawer, for example, or to take laundry out of the dryer. When you squat, your knees and feet should be apart. Lower and raise yourself slowly, and be sure to keep your back straight both going down and coming up.

Lifestyle 149

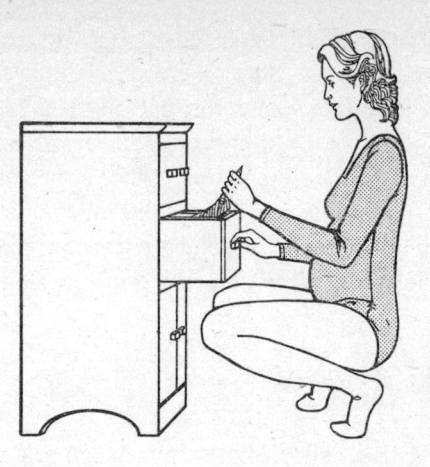

Tailor Sitting

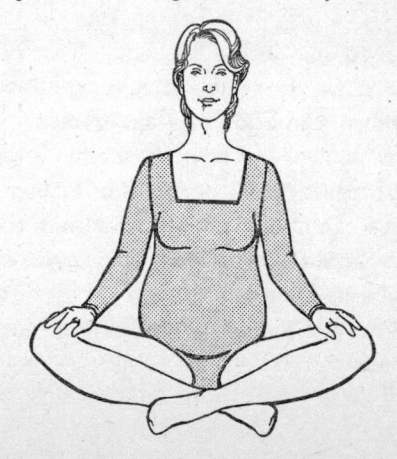

This is another example of a nonexercise that is beneficial. Tailor sitting is recommended during pregnancy because it places the weight of the baby and uterus forward, taking pressure off the back. It also helps limber thigh and pelvic muscles. Sit on the floor and cross your ankles in front of you; straighten your back and lean *slightly* forward with your hands resting on your knees. Be careful not to slouch or lean on the uterus. Tailor sit whenever you have the opportunity—while reading the Sunday paper, snapping green beans, watching television, playing with your toddler.

Kegel Exercise

This is a relatively simple but extremely important exercise that involves tightening and relaxing the pelvic floor muscles. It is named after Dr. Arnold Kegel, a California obstetrician-gynecologist who has done a great deal of research on the function of the pelvic floor. The pelvic floor muscles support the bladder, the uterus, and the bowel, and they are under increased pressure as the uterus enlarges. This is why it is so important to keep these muscles in good tone during pregnancy. If the pelvic floor muscles are weak, their supporting function is impaired and this, in turn, can lead to certain problems, including poor bladder control and possibly uterine prolapse in a subsequent pregnancy or later in life. Weakened pelvic floor muscles can also cause a slackness of the vaginal walls, which can result in decreased pleasure for a woman and a man during intercourse.

The best way to locate the pelvic floor muscles and the action involved in tightening and relaxing them is to stop and start the flow of urine once or twice when you go to the bathroom. This may not be easy at first, but if you practice each time you must urinate, you'll soon get the hang of it. Concentrate on the muscles and the action involved in stopping and starting the flow. Do not use your abdominal or buttock muscles, and do not hold your breath. Once you've learned the technique, you can practice the Kegel exercise anytime, anywhere, and in any position—standing, sitting, or lying down. When doing Kegels, be sure to lift in and up; you should not bear down. Tighten the muscles slowly, hold for a few seconds only, then slowly relax. When you first begin, do two or three Kegels at a time, then increase the number to five at a time. As you become more proficient, try to do Kegels 20 or 30 times a day.

Doing Kegels regularly during pregnancy can also help prepare you for second stage labor, when relaxing the pelvic floor is so important in effectively pushing the baby down and out of the birth canal. Kegels should also be resumed as soon as possible after delivery to help restore muscle tone.

The Sporting Life

If you participated in sports before you became pregnant, you needn't be sidelined now. When pregnancy is progressing normally, a woman can usually continue with most sports in which she has already gained some proficiency. This is not the time, however, to begin learning a sport. Remember, your body is already undergoing a new stress called pregnancy. Even if you are an expert, you should always consult with your physician or nurse-midwife before continuing your favorite sports. She may have sound reason to rule out certain activities in your particular case. In addition, some sports are inadvisable now, including contact sports, water skiing, and scuba diving.

Even when you have your caregiver's okay, there are some common-sense precautions to keep in mind. First of all, pregnancy is not the time to try to win competitions. When you participate in a sport, do it for fun and relaxation. Second, be sensitive to your body and know your limits. Be sure to stop at the first sign of any discomfort, and do not overexert yourself—you should stop and rest before you get fatigued, not after. Do not engage in sports when the weather is hot and humid or when other hazardous conditions exist—bicycling in the rain, for example. Finally, keep in mind that no matter how agile you may be, you are going to become progressively less so, and you will have to adjust your activity to your increasing weight and changing balance. Once a sport becomes uncomfortable or your changing balance increases the risk of falling, the time has come to stop. Pregnancy and play are not mutually exclusive. Just let common sense guide you, and have a good time.

Swimming

When you're pregnant, swimming feels terrific. There's nothing quite like the weightlessness that water provides you with, now that your body is heavier and more awkward. You will feel graceful again. Swimming is an excellent sport; it utilizes many different muscle groups and stimulates circulation too. If you're doing laps, it's important to pace yourself and do them slowly. Remember, you're not in training for the Olympics, so don't overexert yourself. When necessary, stop and rest between laps. Don't try your skill at diving during pregnancy, and don't jump into the water feet first because of the danger of water being forced up into the vagina. Whether or not you're an expert swimmer, you might want to consider taking a prenatal water exercise class. These classes are becoming very popular, and you might try calling your local Y to see if it offers such a program. Doing exercises in the water is just as beneficial as doing them on land and can feel even better.

Bicycle Riding

Pregnancy is not the time to learn to ride a bike, but if you're an experienced cyclist, this is a great form of exercise, especially for the legs. It helps stimulate circulation and respiration too. During pregnancy, it's best to ride a bike with standard handlebars, rather than a racing bike, so that you can sit up straight. Get off and walk the bike whenever you feel tired or must climb a hill. In the summer, avoid cycling in the heat of the day; stick to the cooler early morning or early evening hours. And pay special attention to your balance as your abdomen enlarges.

Tennis

If you played tennis on a regular basis, you can usually continue now. But be careful about overstretching when reaching for a ball, and don't run all over the court after every ball. As your abdomen increases, your balance will shift, and you may find it difficult to compensate. Never play tennis in excessive heat, and be sure to stop before you get fatigued.

Jogging

If you weren't a jogger before pregnancy, don't start jogging now. If you did jog on a regular basis, you can usually continue, but be sure to do your warm-up exercises first. You may already be wearing a good supportive bra, but if not, definitely wear one when jogging. Support hose can be helpful too. As with tennis, don't jog in excessive heat, and be sure to stop before you get fatigued. Remember, it's not how far you jog but the exercise that counts. Keep in mind, too, that there is increased pressure on the bladder during pregnancy and that jogging accentuates this pressure.

Bowling

This is a popular activity for many people, and if it's one that you enjoy, you can continue during pregnancy. Your form, however, will have to be modified as your abdomen increases and your balance changes. Pay attention to your breathing, and take care to avoid quick twists of your body.

Lifestyle

Golf

The walking involved in golf is excellent exercise. Your swing, however, will have to be greatly modified to compensate for your increasing abdomen. This is another sport that should be avoided on hot and humid days.

If you did not participate in sports before you become pregnant, there is one activity that you can do now—walk. Walking is terrific exercise, and a brisk 20- or 30-minute walk each day will pay benefits now and later. Walking is free, convenient, and suitable for just about everyone. And all you need is a sensible pair of shoes.

Travel

Whether your trip is for business or pleasure, across the state or across the country, health professionals agree that you need have no hesitation about traveling during pregnancy, unless you are experiencing complications or have a history of medical problems. Just be sensible and practical—planning ahead even more carefully than you do ordinarily—and you'll be all set, whatever your destination.

Timing

In general, the second trimester is probably the best time to take a pleasure trip. In the first three months of pregnancy, nausea and fatigue may limit your energy and interest. Many women are at their most energetic during the middle months, making it a good time for a holiday. Also, the rate of complications is lowest during this period. During the last trimester, your increasing weight can make you less mobile and more uncomfortable. Toward the end of pregnancy, also, you don't want to be too far from home.

Before making a definite decision, you should discuss your travel plans with your physician or nurse-midwife. There are many factors to consider, even when pregnancy is progressing normally. For example, it's wise to know where you can get good medical care, should you need it. If you are traveling in the United States, ask your caregiver to recommend a doctor or hospital at your destination. If he can't make a recommendation ahead of time, the local medical society should be able to give you a reference on arrival. If you are going abroad, your travel agent may be able to supply you with information on competent medical facilities for each stop of your itinerary. Ask if they know the names of foreign physicians who were trained in the U.S. and who speak English, or if they know how you can obtain such names. Ideally, you should have this information before you leave, but if you don't, be sure to inquire at your hotel or the U.S. consulate when you arrive. More than likely, a medical problem will not arise, but it's best to be prepared just in case.

In addition, ask your caregiver for a medical record card with your blood type and other pertinent information. Discuss any medications, including prenatal vitamins, that you may be taking, and be sure to bring a sufficient supply with you. Ask about remedies for common traveler's ailments, such as upset stomach and diarrhea. Remember, you should not take any medication, either prescription or over-the-counter, without your caregiver's knowledge and approval. If you are considering visiting a foreign country where immunizations are required, it's best to change your plans, since many vaccines are not recommended for use in pregnancy. As a final precaution, find out ahead of time if your health insurance will cover you at your destination in the unlikely event of a medical emergency. And be sure to take your insurance card with you.

Modes of Transportation

Whether you travel by car, plane, bus, or train depends a lot on personal preference and on the distance to be covered. However you go, the important thing to keep in mind is that you should vary your position as frequently as possible. Sitting still for a long period of time impedes circulation, which can cause swelling of the legs and feet, and contribute to varicose veins and other problems. If you are traveling by car, you should plan a rest stop at least once every two hours. Get out of the car and walk around to get your circulation moving. If you're traveling by plane, train, or bus, stand up occasionally and stretch, and walk in the aisle when conditions permit. When you are seated, you can do some simple foot and leg exercises to stimulate circulation: rotate your ankles first clockwise, then counterclockwise; stretch out your legs and flex your feet toward you, then away; place both feet flat on the floor, and move up and down on heels and toes. Be sure to wear comfortable shoes and, whenever possible, keep your legs elevated.

Traveling itself is tiring, and during pregnancy you are going to find it even more so. If you are going by car, you should set a limit on how much distance you cover each day—between 250 and 300 miles is generally recommended, with, remember, frequent rest stops to stretch your legs. There isn't any reason why you can't share some of the driving, as long as you still fit comfortably behind the wheel. Always be sure to wear your seat belt. Buckle it low, well under the abdomen and across the pelvis. The shoulder harness gives extra protection but should not be worn alone.

The main advantage of bus travel is that you don't have to do the driving. You are, however, at the mercy of the bus schedule, so you should check it out in advance to be sure the rest stops are frequent enough. Between stops, remember to stand and stretch occasionally, and to walk in the aisle when conditions permit. A lengthy trip should be broken up with stopovers along the way.

You have more freedom of movement on a train than on a bus, and there's often a snack or restaurant car to provide a change of scene. Trains also have nonsmoking cars, which you should select whenever possible. For an overnight trip, a good investment in comfort is a slumber coach or sleeping compartment. In addition, train travel generally causes less motion sickness than car or bus travel.

A long-distance trip usually means flying. When you travel by plane, be sure to request an aisle seat. This way, you can get up regularly and stretch your legs without inconveniencing anyone. For additional comfort, you

Lifestyle

might want to request a bulkhead or front-row seat. These seats usually have more leg room, which can be an advantage. When you are seated, keep your feet propped on your carry-on bag, and every once in a while, do your leg and foot exercises. Your feet and ankles may swell during the flight from the added air pressure, so don't take off your shoes or you may not be able to get them back on. Be sure to wear your seat belt when the seat belt sign is on. Buckle it low, well under the abdomen.

Many airlines require a medical certificate approving a flight in late pregnancy. Regulations, however, vary from airline to airline. While it isn't wise to travel far from home at this time, if a flight is absolutely necessary, be sure to check with your caregiver and the airline ahead of time. Another thing to keep in mind is that you should fly only in pressurized aircraft during pregnancy, since changes in air pressure can affect the flow of oxygen to the baby.

Although many pregnant women would turn green just thinking about traveling by ship, some find it very pleasant. A sea cruise can be a relaxing way to reach a destination or can be a vacation in itself. It should cause no special problems if you're normally a good sailor. Pregnancy, however, may not be the time to find out how good a sailor you are. If you are planning a vacation cruise, be sure to find out ahead of time what medical facilities are available aboard ship.

Other Travel Tips

Plan your travel wardrobe with comfort in mind. Loose-fitting clothing and low-heeled shoes—the lowest you can comfortably wear—are your best wardrobe bets. Bring at least two pairs of sensible walking shoes so you can alternate their use. If you will be away for several weeks, be sure to pack clothes that will fit as you grow.

Don't take a vacation from proper nutrition—it's just as important when you are away as when you are home. If you are traveling in a foreign country where the safety of the drinking water is suspect, drink bottled water instead. Always specify pasteurized milk or, better yet, bring packets of powdered milk with you. Be wary of raw fruits and vegetables; stick to simple, wholesome foods that have been thoroughly cooked.

When you're out in the sun, cover your head with a hat or a scarf. Body metabolism increases during pregnancy and you're going to feel the heat more. Be sure to drink lots of wholesome liquids to guard against dehydration.

Try to know and anticipate your limits. Alternate periods of sightseeing and other activities with periods of rest. Just relax and enjoy yourself—after all, that's what a vacation is all about.

5. Preparing for Baby

When you first become pregnant, the nine months seem to stretch out so far ahead of you. It's like standing on the shore of an ocean and trying to picture the land on the other side. But somehow the weeks and months slip by, and you're suddenly halfway through your pregnancy or even more. The baby will be here before you know it, and there are many preparations to be made—from buying baby furniture and clothing to choosing a pediatrician and deciding whether to breast- or bottle-feed.

Buying for Baby

Selecting baby furniture and clothing can be both the most enjoyable part of your preparations and the most anxiety-producing. Who doesn't love looking at tiny baby clothes, colorful quilts, stuffed toys, and whimsical mobiles? But now that you are justified in spending hours in the layette department, you may find yourself suffering from an approach-avoidance conflict. Part of you can't wait to get your hands on the luscious little things while part of you hesitates. You may feel a little embarrassed, a little confused, and a little superstitious, as if buying baby items is somehow playing with fate. While not all expectant mothers experience such feelings, many are surprised to find that they do. There's not a lot that can be done about them, except to recognize that they're perfectly normal and that they'll be dispelled once the baby is born. In the meantime, shopping with a friend or relative can help, especially one who is a new mother. She'll not only be able to relate to your feelings, she'll be able to give you valuable advice about your purchases.

The following shopping guide is divided into three categories: furniture and equipment; clothing, bedding, and other cloth items; and drug store items. It is based on the latest consumer information, as well as on my experience and that of other mothers. If you know any new mothers, be sure to speak with them also. They can often provide valuable information, especially on individual brands and stores.

Furniture and Equipment

Safety should be your prime consideration when choosing baby furniture and equipment. Babies are very vulnerable, and what they come in contact with must be as safe as possible. Keep in mind, too, that no matter how well a product is made, it is only safe if it is used correctly.

Crib, Cradle, or Bassinet A newborn can sleep in any number of places, including a crib, a cradle, or a bassinet.

Preparing for Baby

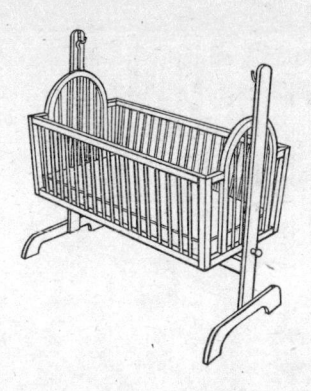

A cradle or bassinet is appealing and provides a cozy place for a tiny baby to sleep. It's only appropriate, however, for the first few months. Once the baby gets bigger and more active, you'll need a roomier and sturdier place for her to sleep. So if you don't buy one at the beginning, you will eventually have to buy a standard-size crib. Parents who live in two-story houses or apartments often find it convenient to keep a cradle, bassinet, or portable crib on the main floor. This way, they don't have to trek up and down the stairs and can keep the baby close by during the day. Portable cribs are smaller and lighter than standard-size cribs, and can be easily folded. Many parents find them great to take on vacations or visits to grandma's. Actually, grandparents often buy their own portable cribs to have on hand when their new grandchildren are brought to visit.

A standard-size crib will probably be the most expensive piece of nursery equipment that you will buy. It is also going to be the most used, so it's wise to buy the best quality that you can afford. All cribs sold in the United States must meet federal safety standards. You can judge the safety of a crib, both standard-size and portable, by checking for the following:

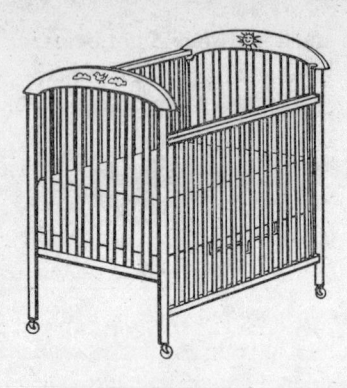

Crib slats must be no more than 2⅜ inches apart. Slats farther apart are dangerous, because a baby's head could get caught between them.

There must be no hazardous cutouts in end or side panels. This is a relatively new regulation, so be sure to check any crib you may be considering for this potential danger. As with slats that are more than 2⅜ inches apart, a baby's head could get caught.

Teething rails must be nontoxic and secure. All wood surfaces must be smooth and free of splinters. All metal hardware must be safe, with no sharp or rough edges.

A dropside must lock at maximum height, and must have safe, secure locking devices that cannot be accidentally released or released by the baby inside the crib.

In addition, the crib mattress must fit snugly. Standard-size cribs usually do not come with mattresses, and you will have to purchase one separately. Be sure the one you buy is the right size for the crib. If you can fit more than two fingers between the mattress and the crib side, the

Preparing for Baby

mattress is too small and should not be used.

Keep all of these safety considerations in mind when you are looking for a crib, and especially if you are considering using a secondhand crib. If you are considering buying a cradle, be sure that the slats are not more than 2⅜ inches apart and that the mattress fits snugly.

Changing Table Not everyone considers a changing table a necessity, but it is the most convenient and comfortable way to change and dress a baby. It's the right height so you don't have to bend over, and all your supplies are close at hand. Changing tables come in a variety of styles, so shop around to see what suits your taste and your pocketbook.

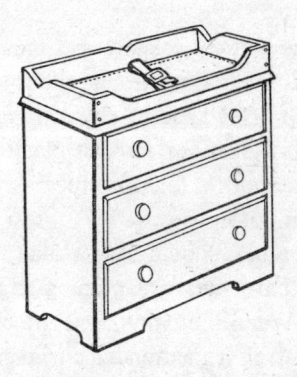

Many cribs come with matching chests that are designed to serve as changing tables. Typically, the chest has three or four drawers and a protective railing around the top, together with a pad and restraining strap. The railing may be part of the chest or it may be mounted separately. Also available are changing kits for adapting a regular chest.

A less expensive type of changing table consists of a

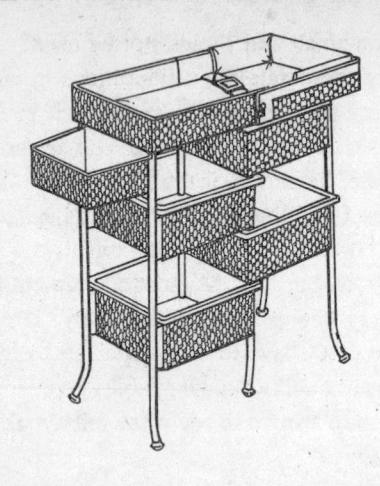

changing surface with open shelves or bins beneath it. It, too, has a protective railing around the top, a pad, and a restraining strap. This type of changing table is usually made of wood, wicker, or molded plastic with tubular steel legs. Some models fold into themselves to take up less space when not in use.

All changing tables should have a pad to provide a soft surface for the baby and a restraining strap to keep the baby in place. When the baby is on the changing table, she should not be left unattended for even a second. It comes as a surprise to many new mothers, but babies often urinate or have bowel movements during diaper changes, especially when you've just removed one diaper and are about to put a clean one underneath. Boys are more likely to get *you* wet. When changing a boy, it's helpful to keep a washcloth or folded cloth diaper over his penis to protect you from an unexpected stream. Don't be fooled into complacency by thinking that he just uri-

Preparing for Baby

nated so he's not going to do it again so soon. You have a 50 percent chance of losing that one!

Baby Bath Your mother probably bathed you in a bathinette, which is a plastic tub on a waist-high stand. Bathinettes are difficult to find nowadays, although they are still being made and usually double as changing tables.

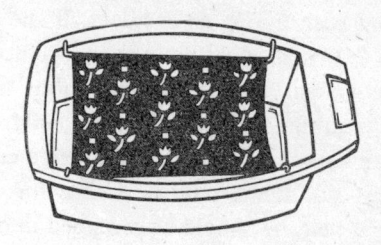

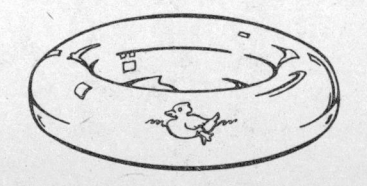

More popular today are conventional baby bathtubs made of molded plastic. They can be used on any waist-high table or counter top so that you don't have to strain your back bending over, which is the main advantage of a bathinette. Many plastic tubs come with different features, including slip-resistant and cushioned bottoms, and detachable hammocks. A hammock cradles and supports the baby, and so gives the parent more hand freedom. Another type of baby bathtub is the inflatable vinyl tub. This, too, helps free the parent's hands because the baby is supported by the soft, rounded sides of the tub. Regardless of what type of tub you use, the cardinal rule when bathing a baby is that she should never be left unattended, not even for a second.

Car Seat A parent's arms are *not* the best or safest place for a baby or child while riding in a car. If the parent is not wearing a seat belt, her body could crush the child against the dashboard or windshield, or against the back of the front seat, during an accident. If she is wearing a seat belt, the child could be torn right out of her grasp during a collision. As of early 1984, more than 40 states had laws requiring babies and young children to be secured in an auto restraint while riding in a car. From the baby's first ride home until he is big enough to use a regular seat belt, he should be strapped into a safe auto restraint every time he is in the car, no matter how short the ride.

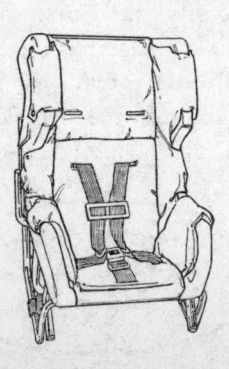

Like cribs, auto restraints must meet federal safety standards. These standards were upgraded several years ago, and all restraints manufactured after January 1, 1981, must withstand actual crash or dynamic testing. When shopping for an auto restraint, look for a label giving the date of manufacture. If you are considering using a secondhand restraint that was manufactured before January 1, 1981, it may or may not be safe. Two organizations—Physicians for Automotive Safety (PAS) and the American Academy of Pediatrics (AAP)—will answer questions about the safety of specific auto restraints. So don't take chances. If you want to know about the safety of a secondhand restraint, write to either of these organizations. Their addresses are: Physicians for Automotive Safety, P.O. Box 208, Rye, New York 10580; American Academy of Pediatrics, Division of Health Education, 1801 Hinman Avenue, Evanston, Illinois 60201. These two organizations also offer publications that contain useful buying information, as well as list brand names and model numbers. The PAS publication is called *Don't Risk Your Child's Life!* and is available for 35¢. The AAP publication is called *A Family Shopping Guide to Infant/Child Automobile Restraints* and a single copy is free. When sending for either of these publications, be sure to include a stamped, self-addressed long white envelope.

There are three types of auto restraints: those made for young babies weighing up to 17 or 20 pounds; those made for older babies and toddlers who can sit up by themselves; and "convertible" restraints, which can be adapted for use with infants as well as older babies and toddlers. The convertible type has become the most common. Infants ride facing rearward in a semireclining position; older babies and toddlers ride facing forward in an upright position.

When considering an auto restraint, be sure that it will fit properly in your car and that the car's lap belts are long enough to secure the restraint. Some restraints come with top anchor or tether straps. An anchor strap provides an extra margin of protection, but if it is not secured or is secured incorrectly, the restraint will *not* be safe. Unless you are certain that you will anchor the strap exactly as directed in the instruction booklet, your baby will be safer in a restraint that doesn't require one. Before buying an auto restraint, ask to see the instruction booklet, and, if possible, try out the restraint in your car first. This way, you can be sure the restraint fits properly. Also consider the baby's comfort and how easy a restraint is to use. In their April 1982 issue, *Consumer Reports* evaluated many brands and styles of auto restraints for safety, comfort, and ease of installation and use. You might want to check out their report at your local library or write to Consumers Union for a reprint order form. Their address is 256 Washington Street, Mount Vernon, New York 10553.

Front and Back Carriers The soft front carrier that is worn by the parent has become a very popular way to

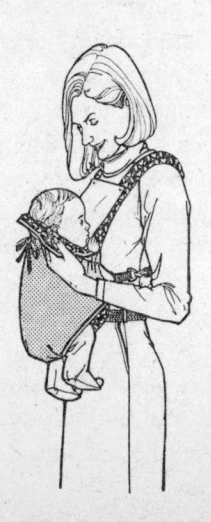

Preparing for Baby

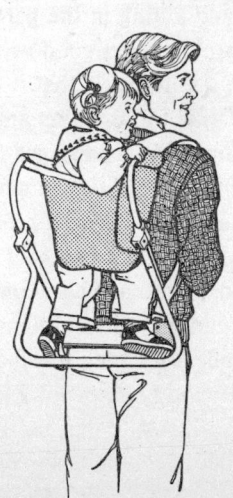

tote a baby, both indoors and out. Nearly anywhere you go, you're likely to see an infant comfortably nestled against his parent's chest in one of these carriers. Babies love the movement and close body contact, and parents find the carriers very convenient because they leave their hands relatively free. Front carriers are designed for use with young babies up to about six months old, although some can be adapted for use with an older baby. These carriers are made in a variety of fabrics, and when selecting one, you should consider the season in which your baby will be arriving. Your principal considerations, however, should be sturdy construction, comfort, and ease in putting the carrier on and taking it off. Be sure to choose one that provides good head and neck support for the baby and that has wide, well-padded shoulder straps for your comfort. The best way to see if a carrier is easy to get on and off by yourself is to try it out in the store. If a large doll is available, use it to see how easy it is to get the baby in and out of the carrier.

Once a baby can sit up well by herself, she'll be happier in a back carrier. This will give her more freedom of movement and a better view. Back carriers have tubular aluminum frames and fabric seats. Again, you'll want to look for sturdy construction and comfort features for you and the baby, as well as ease in getting the carrier on and off. Be sure the leg holes are not constrictive and that there is enough room for the baby's legs to hang down in front rather than to the sides. Shoulder straps should be wide and well-cushioned, and the front of the frame or top rail should be padded and covered with fabric. Another essential is a safety waist belt, which should always be used.

Carriage Whether or not you buy a carriage will depend on your budget and your lifestyle. If you plan to do a lot of walking and sitting in the park while your baby is tiny, you will probably get good use out of a carriage. The advantage of a carriage is that it usually provides a more comfortable ride for an infant and better protection against the elements. Most carriages fold for storage or for transporting in a car. But even when folded, they're not exactly tiny, and this can be a problem if you live in a small apartment or have a compact car. Carriages, of course, have hoods, but many also come with detachable windscreens that can provide additional protection when necessary. (I found this screen invaluable when walking on our extremely windy boulevard.) When your baby is fussy, you may find rocking him gently or wheeling him in the carriage inside your apartment or house to be helpful.

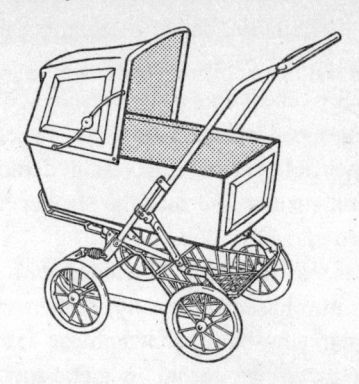

There are basically two types of carriages: those that convert to strollers and those that don't. Usually those that convert will be more expensive, but then you won't have to buy a stroller, unless you want one that's compact and lightweight. Carriages that convert usually form heavier strollers, because the base that's used is the same as for the carriage.

If you are considering buying a carriage, keep the following points in mind when shopping:

The carriage should be stable and difficult to tip.

The brakes should lock tightly and be convenient to apply and release. Most carriages have brakes on two wheels, but some have them on four wheels for additional safety. The wheels should be heavy and sturdy.

The carriage should have very secure locking devices to prevent accidental collapse. There should be no sharp edges or scissorlike mechanisms.

If there is a sit-up back rest, it should give firm support.

Check the height of the handle by taking the carriage on a stroll through the store. Some tall parents prefer carriages with higher handles. Be sure the carriage isn't too heavy for you to push and maneuver comfortably. Keep in mind that a spring-suspension system gives a smoother ride.

Have a salesperson demonstrate how the carriage folds. If it's a convertible carriage, have him demonstrate how it sets up as a stroller. Be sure the stroller portion has a waist-and-crotch safety belt.

Usually, a mattress is not included with the carriage and must be purchased separately. Some carriages come with metal carrying baskets, which are very handy for packages. If a carriage doesn't, a metal tray that fits between the four wheels can usually be bought separately. A carriage can tip easily, and you should never hang a pocketbook or shopping bag from the handle. You should also avoid putting packages inside the carriage, as this also can upset the balance. Once your baby can sit up, you will have to buy a zipper-style harness to keep him secured in the carriage. Remember, too, that carriages are intended for infants. When a baby becomes heavier and more active, he should be in a stroller.

Stroller There are so many brands and models of strollers that the task of choosing one might seem impossible. But there are basically only three categories of strollers: conventional, compact, and a relatively new hybrid called convenience. A conventional stroller usually offers many comfort features, including thick foam padding, a multi-position back, a canopy, a windscreen, and a boot. A compact stroller is lightweight, easy to fold and store, and often has umbrellalike handles. A convenience stroller incorporates some of the comforts of a conventional stroller, but it is more compact, lighter in weight, and easier to fold.

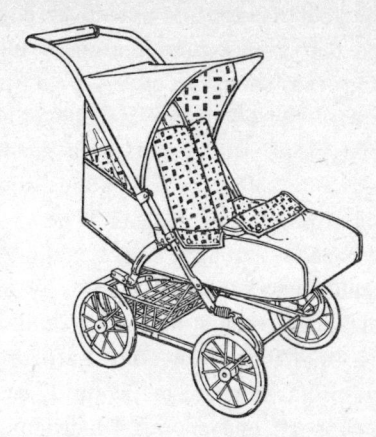

When choosing a stroller, you must give careful thought to what you will be using a stroller for and when you will begin using it. If you want to start using a stroller soon after your baby is born, you will need one that offers carriagelike qualities. The stroller must have a fully reclining back and sides that are high enough to keep the baby from falling out, and it must have a soft, well-padded interior for comfort and protection. Canopy, windscreen, and boot accessories are also important for use when weather conditions dictate. And you should select a stroller that provides the smoothest ride possible. If you don't plan to start using a stroller until your baby is three or four months old, you usually do not need one with a fully reclining back, although this does make a stroller more versatile.

If you plan to keep the stroller in the trunk of your car for an occasional trip to the shopping center or if you'll be using public transportation, you should consider getting a stroller that's easy to open and close and that's relatively light and compact. If you'll be doing the majority of your baby transportation in the stroller—taking walks daily, grocery shopping, etc.—you'll want to select the highest quality stroller that your budget allows.

Whatever type of stroller suits your needs and your baby's needs best, safety considerations should be uppermost in your purchasing decision. The stroller should have a wide base for stability; a back that doesn't tip the stroller's balance when the back is in its lowest position; a sturdy waist-and-crotch strap (which should always be used); brakes that lock firmly; no sharp or protruding edges or scissorlike mechanisms; a sturdy seat that provides good support; and enough headroom for growth when the canopy is up. When shopping for a stroller, look for the safety approved label of the Juvenile Products Manufacturers Association (JPMA). This label means that the stroller was manufactured and tested to meet strict safety standards.

In addition to safety considerations, comfort and convenience features are also important when selecting a stroller. Double wheels and balloon wheels give a smoother ride, and swivel front wheels allow you to maneuver the stroller more easily, particularly up and down curbs. A footrest that comes in contact with the baby's feet will make him more comfortable. Other convenience features include utility baskets and stroller bags for carrying small packages and baby items. Stroller bags, however, must be positioned correctly or they'll upset the stroller's balance. For the same reason, you should never hang shopping bags or pocketbooks from the handle or handles. If you buy a vinyl-backed stroller, you may want to purchase a special stroller seat cover. It makes the seat more

Preparing for Baby

comfortable for the baby and, especially in summer, helps keep him from perspiring because of the vinyl. You can also make your own cover quite easily, or just use a soft terry towel.

Baby Seat Many parents find baby seats a convenient piece of equipment for home, visiting, and travel. Most baby seats are made of molded plastic with padded inserts, and the seats usually adjust to two or three different angles. A newer type of baby seat is a sturdy cloth stretched over a metal frame. This type stays at one angle, but it's an angle babies seem to enjoy.

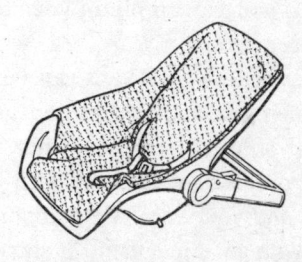

You can think of a baby seat as an extra pair of hands. It can be used soon after your baby is born and is a convenient way to keep her near you, as well as to give her a change of scenery from the crib. We kept our babies in the center of the table during meals. It made them feel part of the family, since they were at eye level and in the midst of the activity, and we were able to watch and tend them while we ate.

When selecting a baby seat, be sure it has a wide base for stability, a nonskid bottom surface, and a sturdy waist-and-crotch strap. Check how many angles the seat can be adjusted to, and be sure the seat locks securely at each angle.

While baby seats are great parents' helpers, they must be used correctly to avoid accidents. Never put a baby seat near the edge of any high surface or on a slippery surface, such as a glass tabletop. Whenever the seat is being used on any off-the-floor surface, you must always be within arms' reach of the baby, and she should never be left unattended, not even for a second. Always be sure to secure the baby in the seat with the waist-and-crotch strap. Keep in mind, too, that these seats are designed for young babies. Once a baby becomes bigger and more active, she has outgrown the seat.

Play Yard If you have room in your home, you may want to consider getting a play yard, which is the new name for a playpen. A play yard can be helpful during those times when you can't keep a constant eye on your baby and need a safe place to put her. If you have a backyard or patio, a play yard can also be put to good use when you and your baby are outdoors. A play yard must be used with good judgment. It should not be overused or used to confine a baby for long periods of time.

Most play yards made today have mesh sides, although those with wood slats are still available. If you choose

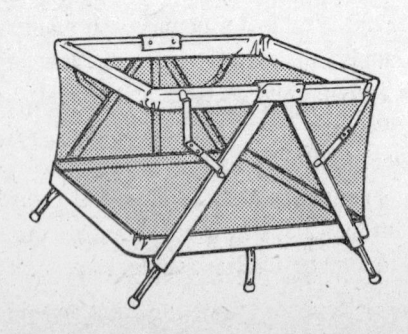

Preparing for Baby

one with slats, be sure the slats are no more than 2⅜ inches apart and that the wood is smooth and free of splinters. With a mesh play yard, you must be certain that the netting has a very tiny weave. The openings in the mesh must be so small that the baby's fingers or toes, or buttons on her clothes, will not get caught. Never buy a play yard with large mesh openings—they are dangerous. Pay special attention to this if you are considering buying a secondhand play yard. Be sure the play yard you select has a strong railing and floor; no sharp edges, points, or protrusions; and secure locking devices to prevent scissoring. When shopping for a play yard, look for the JPMA safety approved label. As with strollers, this label means that the play yard has been manufactured and tested to meet strict safety standards.

Play yards come in two shapes: square and rectangular. Square or full-size play yards are roomier and usually measure 36 inches × 36 inches, although some are a little bit bigger. Rectangular play yards are designed to fit through a doorway. They do not provide as much space for a baby as a full-size play yard, but they are quite portable and may be good if space is a problem for you. Some rectangular play yards have adjustable legs so that they can also be used as portable cribs. There is a very important safety precaution to keep in mind whenever you use a mesh-sided portable crib or any mesh-sided play yard, either full-size or rectangular: Never leave your baby in it with a dropside down. When it is down, the mesh forms a loose pocket that leaves a gap between the edge of the floorboard and the mesh side. An infant or young child may roll or fall into the gap, become trapped, and suffocate. Keep in mind, too, that whenever your baby is in a play yard, you should always keep her in view.

If you do decide to get a play yard, it is not something that you will need immediately after birth, so it isn't necessary to buy one ahead of time, unless you see a good sale. But if someone asks what he or she can get you as a baby gift, a play yard is an item to keep in mind—provided, of course, that the person can afford it.

High Chair You won't be using a high chair until your baby is about six months old. High chairs either are made of wood or have steel frames with cushioned seats and backs. Whichever style you may decide upon, be sure to check for the following safety features: wide-stance legs for stability; no sharp edges or points, or places that can pinch tiny fingers; a tray that locks securely; and a safety belt that is composed of a waist-and-crotch strap. The safety belt should be securely attached to the chair; be sure that it is *not* attached to the tray. High chairs also come with JPMA certification, so when it's time for you to begin shopping, look for ones displaying the JPMA

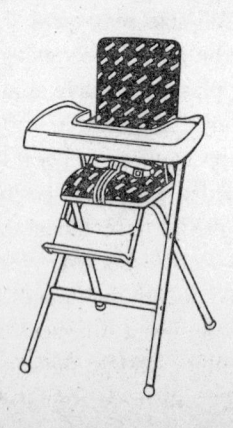

Preparing for Baby

label. When considering different high chairs, test how the trays move in and out. The easier a tray is to operate, the easier your life will be. A roomy feeding tray, especially one that wraps around the sides of the chair, is desirable, as is a tray with raised edges to contain spills. For baby's comfort, look for well-padded cushions and an adjustable footrest. When your baby is in his high chair, he should always be secured with the waist-and-crotch strap. This will keep him seated in the chair and keep him from sliding out under the tray.

Clothing, Bedding, and Other Cloth Items

When you go shopping for the layette, you may be given a list of "essential" items and how much to buy. While such a list can be helpful as a preliminary guide to the world of the layette, only you can judge what and how much you will need. This will depend on many factors, including your budget, whether you have clothes from other children or hand-me-downs from friends, the season in which your baby will be arriving, and how often you plan to do the laundry. You may want to be a bit conservative at first, waiting to see what you receive as gifts and what types of clothes you prefer to use.

Manufacturers size infant clothing several ways: by weight, by age and weight, by height, and by age. Generally, you should use your baby's weight or height as a gauge in selecting the right size. Expectant mothers are often advised not to buy too much in the smallest size. It is true that babies outgrow their clothes quickly, but how much use you'll get out of a small-size garment depends on the size of your baby at birth. My own son weighed 6 pounds, 10 ounces, and the two small stretchies I bought lasted him for several months, and I wished that I had more. Of course, if your baby weighs 9 pounds at birth, he won't be wearing a small size for very long. Before buying baby items, be sure to ask about the store's exchange and return policy. Many stores will let you exchange unopened packages, even if you bought the items months in advance.

Undershirts These are an essential baby item and you will need a good supply. Undershirts are available with short sleeves, long sleeves, and no sleeves, and come in wrap and pullover styles. Some mothers find wrap styles easiest to put on a newborn, but others find it just as easy to use pullover shirts. Be sure that the pullover shirts you buy have expandable or lap shoulder necks. Undershirts come not only in basic white but also in pastels and nursery prints. A summer baby can live in a shirt and diaper, except for special occasions, so if your baby will be arriving in warm weather, you may want to buy a dozen shirts. For other seasons, you may want to start out with six—depending, of course, on how often you plan to do the laundry. The salesperson may suggest that you skip the smallest size and buy the next size up. Again, this depends on the size of your baby or how much you care about the shirt fitting well. If you do buy some in the smallest size, be sure you have the option of exchanging unopened packages in case you find that you prefer the larger size.

Diapers If you plan to use disposable diapers, you may want to buy a small box of several different brands to see which one you like best. Once you do decide, it's most

Preparing for Baby

economical to buy the largest size box. Cloth diapers come in three different fabrics: bird's-eye, flannel, and gauze. Gauze is less absorbent and durable than flannel and bird's-eye but has the advantage of being lighter, cooler, and faster-drying. Gauze is often recommended for warm-weather use. If you plan to use cloth diapers, you will need 3 or 4 dozen if you launder them yourself and 1 dozen to supplement a diaper service. You will also have to buy several pairs of vinyl pants. These aren't necessary if you use disposables, which have waterproof coverings. If you do use disposables, you should still have some cloth diapers on hand. They're good to use as burping cloths, for wiping baby drool, and for similar clean-up jobs.

Stretchies These all-in-one coveralls have become a basic baby item for day and night wear. They typically have snaps which extend down one or two legs to make dressing and diapering easier. Stretchies are common baby gifts, so you may not want to overbuy. Also, if your baby will be born in summer, you may not need stretchies until the fall. A happy medium might be to buy four or five until you see how big your baby is, what you receive as gifts, and how the laundry goes. Don't open all the packages so that you can exchange them if you find that you need a different size or color. Coveralls are available in nonstretch fabrics too.

Gowns These are another baby staple. They are long and loose and typically have mitten-style sleeves and drawstring bottoms. Gowns usually come in one size only, but they're generally fairly big on the newborn and can be worn for some time. My son was still wearing them at four months, without the drawstring. Gowns are easy to put on and allow easy access to the diaper area. The only problem is that when you hold the baby, the gown tends to ride up and the baby's feet begin to stick out through the bottom. You may want to start out with two gowns until you see what you like to use.

Kimonos and Sacques Kimonos are used to top an undershirt and diaper when a little extra warmth is needed. Sacques, which are front-closing smocks, serve a similar function and also give the baby a more dressed look.

Sweaters Buy weights that will be appropriate for the season in which your baby will be born. If it's summer, one or two lightweight sweaters should be sufficient. For other seasons, you will want a couple of sweaters in different weights. You may want to use a lightweight one indoors and a heavier one outdoors.

Bunting or Pram Suit If your baby arrives in cold weather, you will need a bunting or a pram suit for outings. A bunting is a hooded, sleeved bag made in a heavyweight fabric. A pram suit is hooded, zippers up the front, and has arms, legs, and feet. Both come with mittens, which may or may not be detachable.

Receiving Blankets These small, lightweight blankets are used not only as a cover in crib or carriage but also as a wrap when the baby is out of bed. Receiving blankets are the perfect size for swaddling, which most newborns like. Three should be sufficient.

Crib Blankets These usually come in two types: thermal and fleece. Thermal blankets provide warmth without weight; fleece blankets are heavier and are good for cool weather. Depending on the season in which your baby will arrive and on the climate you live in, you may want to consider getting two lightweight blankets and one heavy

Preparing for Baby

one. Crib quilts are also available, and many parents like the style that can be zippered and used as a bunting for outings.

Crib Sheets Fitted sheets come in bassinet/carriage, portable crib, and standard crib sizes. They're available in a variety of colors and patterns, are made of either 100 percent cotton or cotton/polyester blends, and are either woven or knitted. Three or four fitted crib sheets should be sufficient.

Crib Bumpers These provide a soft buffer between the baby and the slats of the crib. Look for ones that are sturdily made and well padded. They should go all around the inside of the crib and be secured with at least six ties or snaps. Bumpers are also available for cradles.

Mattress Pad Even though your crib mattress will probably be moisture-proof, you should still protect it with a waterproof covering. One good choice is a flannel-back rubber mattress pad, which allows some air to circulate. Two of these should be enough.

Lap Pads These are smaller versions of the above that you can put on your lap when feeding or holding your baby to protect your clothes (diapers often leak!). Many mothers also use them as changing pads when out shopping or at a friend's house. You might want to buy two or three until you see how much you use them.

Baby Towels and Washcloths Towels made especially for babies aren't a necessity, but they *are* very soft and absorbent. Especially handy are hooded baby towels. The hood keeps the baby's head warm, absorbs some of the water, and sort of anchors the towel. Two or three baby towels should be fine. The advantages of baby washcloths are that they are softer and a little thinner than regular ones. They're also smaller and therefore easier to use. If you plan to use them strictly for bathing, two should be sufficient. If you think you'll use them for other clean-ups, get a few more.

Drug Store Items

In preparation for your baby's homecoming, you ought to have certain drug store items on hand. These include solid or liquid baby soap, and baby shampoo; baby lotion, powder, or cornstarch; diaper rash ointment; sterile cotton or balls for dabbing and cleaning; blunt-end baby nail scissors; a rectal thermometer; petroleum jelly, which is used to lubricate the thermometer before insertion, and also to protect the diaper area against wetness and the baby's face against wind; and alcohol, which is used to clean the umbilical stump and to clean the thermometer. You may also want to buy one or two pacifiers. It's helpful to have a method other than pacing and rocking to try and calm a baby at three A.M.

You'll be thankful to have one or two good baby books to consult when you want to know how to sterilize a bottle or when to expect your baby's first smile. Some suggested readings are given in the bibliography. Check them out at your local bookstore and see which ones look best to you.

Once you have the essentials in the house, you can heave a huge sigh of relief. Now the baby can arrive whenever he's ready without catching you unprepared. You can congratulate him on having such efficient, organized, and loving parents, who have selected baby items with his safety and comfort uppermost in mind.

Breast or Bottle?

One of the most important decisions you will be making is whether you will breastfeed or bottle-feed. This is not to say that you can't change your mind, but there are many factors to consider, and pregnancy is when you will have time to weigh them all. If you are considering nursing your baby, you have a lot of company. Breastfeeding is definitely on the increase. Between 1971 and 1982, the number of women who chose to breastfeed more than doubled—from about 25 percent to nearly 62 percent, according to a study conducted by Ross Laboratories. More women are choosing to breastfeed because of the nutritional and emotional benefits that nursing provides. Breastfeeding has also been endorsed as the preferred feeding method by many major health organizations, including the American Academy of Pediatrics, the American College of Obstetricians and Gynecologists, and the American Medical Association.

Breastfeeding

The fact is that no food is as nutritionally perfect for an infant as her mother's milk. While commercial infant formulas closely resemble mother's milk, its unique composition cannot be duplicated. Because of its composition, breast milk is very easy for a baby to digest, and her body utilizes nearly all of it. When you nurse your baby, you are also providing her with important immunological protection. Both colostrum, which will nourish the baby for the first few days of life, and mature breast milk contain antibodies which help the baby fight infection. Studies show that breastfed babies experience far fewer respiratory and gastrointestinal illnesses than bottle-fed babies. In addition, because breast milk is designed specifically for the human baby, no baby will be allergic to it. This is an important consideration, especially if you have a family history of allergies. There is also some evidence that breastfeeding can help protect a baby from allergies later in life.

Generally, breastfed babies are less likely to be overweight. A nursing mother can't measure how much milk her baby is taking, and it's up to him to decide when he's had enough. When a mother bottle-feeds, there is a tendency to coax the baby to finish the bottle, and this, in turn, may lead to overfeeding. "I tried so hard not to worry about how much formula the baby was taking," says one mother. "But the ounces were clearly marked on the bottle, and it's so hard not to feel that you want him to take just a little more." In fact, however, it's better if the baby doesn't quite finish the bottle because then you know he's had enough. When a baby is consistently draining his bottles on his own, it is time to add more formula.

Many experts also believe that breastfeeding contributes to the sound development of the baby's jaw and facial muscles. This is because of the vigorous work involved with nursing. The baby must literally milk the breast by rhythmically squeezing the areola, the dark area surrounding the nipple, with her gums.

Preparing for Baby

Nursing also provides many benefits for the mother. When your baby suckles at the breast, the hormone oxytocin is released into your bloodstream. This hormone causes the uterus to contract, and if you can nurse your baby right after delivery, the uterine contractions can help speed expulsion of the placenta. Nursing right after birth can also help reduce the possibility of postpartum hemorrhage. In addition, the contractions brought about by nursing help the uterus return more quickly to its pre-pregnant size. During the early days of breastfeeding, most mothers experience uterine cramps when they nurse their babies. These so-called afterpains are concrete signs that the uterus is contracting and getting smaller.

Another advantage of breastfeeding is that it can help you return more quickly to your pre-pregnancy weight. During pregnancy, the body stores extra fat in preparation for milk production, and it does this whether you plan to breastfeed or not. While you must consume about 500 extra calories each day when you nurse, nursing itself burns up approximately 900 calories a day. What this means is that you will steadily shed the fat stores that were laid down during pregnancy. Women who bottle-feed often find it harder to lose these extra pounds.

The convenience of breastfeeding cannot be overestimated. The milk is always ready and at the right temperature. There is no formula to prepare, no bottles and nipples to sterilize, and no waiting period while the baby's meal is being warmed. A mother who breastfed one baby and bottle-fed another attests to the convenience: "For me, the worst part of bottle-feeding was warming the bottle for the middle-of-the-night feeding. Holding a crying and hungry baby, the five or ten minutes it took to warm the bottle seemed interminable. When I breastfed, I picked up the baby when he cried, put him to my breast, and he was quiet and happy, as was I."

One more advantage for the mother is that in general, breastfeeding requires only one arm, leaving the other arm free to stroke the baby, to read a book, to hug or to read to an older child, or to talk on the telephone.

It's unfortunate that in our society many women have little if any exposure to breastfeeding. Nursing mothers are just not as common a sight in this country as they are in others. "I had never, ever, seen someone breastfeed before my daughter was born," says one mother who nursed her baby for six months. Another mother, who traveled to Mexico during her pregnancy, tells this story: "We were riding on a crowded local bus when a mother who was sitting across from me with her baby took out a cloth diaper and opened it up. I kept looking at her, wondering how on earth she was going to change her baby on the bus, when she put one corner of the diaper in her mouth, put the baby next to her breast, and covered him with the diaper. She had formed a kind of tent with the diaper to give her privacy while she nursed. Here I was, in my seventh month, planning to breastfeed, and it took at least five minutes for it to dawn on me what this woman was doing."

If you have not had the opportunity to know and observe a nursing mother, you may find it harder to decide what you want to do, and it may help to go to a La Leche League meeting. La Leche League is an international organization dedicated to the support of nursing mothers and to the dissemination of breastfeeding information. The League has local chapters throughout the country which hold regular meetings that pregnant women and

Preparing for Baby

nursing mothers attend. You will not only have the opportunity to ask questions and pick up a lot of helpful information, you will also be able to observe mothers nursing their babies. Many women who sincerely want to breastfeed are afraid that they will be embarrassed about it. It is difficult to assuage such fears, unless you either observe a mother nursing—so you can see how natural and unrevealing it is—or do it yourself. "I was desperately afraid of nursing in front of other people, because I thought my breasts would show," says one new mother. "But I practiced in front of a mirror and realized that I could nurse very discreetly. The more casual I felt about nursing, the better I felt." Of course, other people can make you uncomfortable either through their own unease with the situation or because of rude comments. The more at ease you are, however, the more comfortable they will be too.

Many men feel uncomfortable at first with the idea of their wives breastfeeding in front of others, but this usually passes when they see how discreetly a baby can be nursed. A father's support and encouragement are essential if breastfeeding is to be successful, and it's important that you and your husband discuss your feelings about nursing ahead of time. Your husband—or you perhaps—may have conflicting feelings about the sexual vs. nursing function of the breasts. Sometimes, a man may be very possessive of his wife's body and just can't get used to the idea of sharing it. More often than not, however, if a man has reservations about breastfeeding, it's because he knows so little about it. Most men, after all, have even less exposure to breastfeeding than women. Many La Leche League chapters offer special sessions for fathers, and your husband may find it very helpful to attend one. To see if there's a League chapter near you, look in your telephone directory or contact the national headquarters—its address is given on page 289. You'll also find several suggested readings in the bibliography. The best way to get breastfeeding off to a good start is to learn as much about it as you can ahead of time—through reading and by speaking with nursing parents.

Bottle-feeding

Even if you do decide to nurse your baby, chances are that you will eventually be giving her a bottle. Many nursing mothers wean their babies from breast to bottle at about six months, if not before. And some women choose to bottle-feed exclusively for a variety of reasons.

Cow's milk forms the basis for most commercial infant formulas, and the milk is processed so that it approximates human milk. Many pediatricians recommend that a bottle-fed baby be given formula for the entire first year. Some doctors, however, believe that whole cow's milk may be acceptable *after* six months. If you do decide to bottle-feed or if you wean your baby from breast to bottle, your pediatrician will recommend a formula for you to use.

Commercial formula is available in two basic types: concentrated and ready-to-use. Concentrated formula comes in powdered and liquid form. This type of formula must be diluted with water. Be sure to read the label carefully and to follow the instructions exactly. It's essential that the correct amount of water be mixed with

Preparing for Baby

the correct amount of formula. Ready-to-use formula comes in 32-ounce cans, 8-ounce six-packs, and in individual disposable baby bottles. The more convenient a formula is to use, the more expensive it will be. Concentrated powdered formula usually costs the least and ready-to-use formula in disposable bottles the most. These are great for travel, and also for middle-of-the-night feedings if your pocketbook can stand it. You don't have to warm a bottle—all you do is open a disposable bottle and attach a collar and nipple.

If you plan to bottle-feed exclusively, you should have at least six bottles and nipples. Baby bottles come in plastic or glass and in 4- and 8-ounce sizes. Also available are disposable bottles. These are presterilized plastic containers that fit inside a holder. You will also need a bottle brush and a nipple brush. These are really essential to keep your equipment clean. You should speak with your baby's doctor about sterilizing equipment. Some doctors advise sterilizing bottles and nipples for the first few months. Others believe that a thorough scrubbing and rinsing are sufficient.

The feelings of warmth and security that a baby gets when she's being fed are as important as the nutritional value of the meal, and a bottle-fed baby should always be held for a feeding. Not only is propping a bottle potentially unsafe, the important love component will be missing. Remember to take your cues from your baby as to when she's had enough, and don't try to coax her to finish every last drop. A fat baby is not necessarily a healthy baby. There is some evidence that obesity in infancy can lead to weight problems in adulthood. Whether or not this is true, a fat baby will be a less active baby and may develop a habit of overeating that is hard to break.

One of the nicest aspects of bottle-feeding is that a father can participate from the very beginning. Fathers enjoy the closeness they feel to their babies during feeding times, and mothers appreciate the relief.

Combining Bottle-feeding and Breastfeeding

While most expectant mothers think of the feeding issue as an either/or proposition, it doesn't have to be. Breastfeeding and bottle-feeding can be successfully combined. If you think you may want to combine the methods, you will have to breastfeed exclusively until your milk supply is well established, which usually takes four to six weeks. In fact, even if you decide to bottle-feed exclusively, nursing for even a month or two will help give your baby important immunological protection. Once your milk supply is well established, you can try to supplement one daily feeding. Once your baby has adjusted to taking a bottle for this feeding and your body has adjusted to making that much less milk, you can try to supplement another feeding. This is often the method that nursing mothers use when they are ready to return to work. Many nurse in the morning and evening and have their child's caretaker supplement with formula or expressed breast milk during the day. Some women adjust easily to this type of schedule, while others find they must express milk in the middle of the day to keep themselves comfortable or to keep up their milk supply.

Even if you decide to breastfeed exclusively, you may

Preparing for Baby

feel psychologically more free if you know that a sitter can give the baby a bottle when you go out. There isn't any reason why a supplementary bottle can't be given once or twice a week after the milk supply is well established. Many nursing mothers have their husbands give the baby a bottle during the nighttime feeding on the weekends so that they can get some rest.

In deciding to combine feeding methods, either frequently or infrequently, you should be aware that occasionally a baby will decide for himself what he wants when he has had both the breast and a bottle. Some breastfed babies start to refuse the breast because nursing from a bottle is so much easier. And some breastfed babies won't take a bottle, no matter how much you want them to. When the baby thwarts your plans, it can be very frustrating.

In making a decision about which feeding method to use, the most important consideration is what you think is best for you and your baby. Whether you decide to breast- or bottle-feed, or to combine the two, you will need time, patience, and support. But that goes for all aspects of baby care.

Choosing a Pediatrician

Choosing a pediatrician may seem like an unnecessary task while you are pregnant, but it is actually crucial to your peace of mind and to your baby's health. You won't have the time to interview prospective pediatricians after your baby is born and a medical problem could arise.

That's not the time to start looking. Although many first-time mothers don't realize it, you may feel like consulting your baby's doctor for any number of reasons before it's time for the initial checkup, which is usually scheduled for about ten days after birth. New mothers call their pediatricians for simple questions like "Should I sterilize the bottles?" or "Should I give my baby a pacifier?" as well as for more serious concerns about fever or prolonged crying.

One expectant mother just didn't understand the usefulness of choosing her baby's doctor ahead of time, since a pediatrician on staff at the hospital could do the comprehensive newborn exam. She thought she'd have enough time to consider pediatricians when she and the baby came home. She regretted her decision afterward. "My son became slightly jaundiced after birth," she explains, "and was released from the hospital on the condition that I bring him back every day for a bilirubin count until the problem cleared up. I had the option of taking him to my pediatrician, but, of course, I didn't have one. I chose one immediately, but he preferred not to get involved until the jaundice cleared up, since he hadn't examined the baby in the hospital. It meant that every day for a week I had to trek to the hospital in rush-hour traffic and to wait 45 minutes for the test results. It was an exhausting way to begin new parenthood."

Once your baby is born, you will get to know and rely on your pediatrician more than on any doctor you have ever used before. Because of the significant role that she will play in your life and in your baby's, it is essential that you find a pediatrician in whom you have confidence, who shares your feelings about child-rearing, and whose

Preparing for Baby

personality meshes with yours and your child's. If you have the typical concerns of new parents and if your baby has one or more illnesses during the first year, you will be calling and visiting your pediatrician more than you can imagine. You don't want to be in a position of hesitating to call with a question or dreading to take your baby in for checkups because you feel uncomfortable with the doctor you've chosen. So be sure to allow yourself sufficient time during pregnancy to find the pediatrician that's right for you.

You can begin your search by speaking with friends, relatives, and co-workers who have young children. Ask who their pediatricians are and what they like and dislike about them. When listening to an opinion, keep in mind the personality of the person who is giving it. Different parents look for different qualities in their pediatricians. You will certainly want to know if a doctor is easy to reach, especially in an emergency, and if he is sensitive and responsive to the child and to the parents' questions and concerns. If you plan to breastfeed, you should also ask if a doctor is supportive of nursing. Office location is another important consideration. If you do not have access to a car or to good public transportation, you should try to find a doctor within walking distance. Even if you do have a car or a bus stop right outside your door, proximity is a plus. You don't want to have to spend an extra 30 minutes in traveling time when an ill baby has to be seen by the doctor. On the other hand, if it's a choice between an excellent pediatrician who is 15 minutes away and a mediocre one who is next door, the 15-minute trip will be well worth it. Another thing to keep in mind is whether you want a pediatrician who is in solo or group practice. If a doctor practices alone, she will probably get to know you and your baby quite well. There will be times, however, when she will be unavailable. The advantage to group practice is that someone is usually on call 24 hours a day, seven days a week. This can mean a speedy response when you are most desperate. (Babies and children have a tendency to become unbearably ill after office hours, in the middle of the night, and on Sunday.) With a group practice, you can often choose one pediatrician whom you will see regularly.

In addition to getting recommendations from parents, you might also speak with your physician, nurse-midwife, childbirth educator, or a local La Leche League leader about prospective pediatricians. Once you've narrowed down the choices to two or three candidates, make an appointment to visit each. Most pediatricians are used to consultations with expectant parents. Some charge a fee; others don't. It's possible that you really won't know how much you like a particular doctor until you have to deal with her as a new mother, but you will have some idea of whom you like and don't like from these interviews. When you call for an appointment, ask how long the doctor usually allots for a consultation so you'll know how much time you'll have and can ask your most important questions first. Be sure to prepare your questions ahead of time; write them out and bring the written questions with you. The following are some of the more important areas that should be covered:

1. If the doctor is in group practice, will you be seeing her regularly? Is a physician on call 24 hours a day, seven days a week, to handle emergency situations?

Preparing for Baby

If a doctor is in solo practice, who covers for her when she is unavailable? How are emergencies handled?

2. What are the doctor's hospital affiliations? Does he have privileges at the hospital where you plan to deliver? Will he be able to do the comprehensive newborn exam?

3. Does the doctor have a special phone-in time when parents can call and ask her nonemergency questions? How are routine calls normally handled? Does the doctor provide any printed material for new parents, such as instructions on baby care or guidelines on development?

4. How often does the doctor schedule well-baby checkups? Some doctors schedule them once a month for the first six months, then every other month for the second six months. Other doctors schedule them once a month for the entire first year.

5. Are any special provisions made for well-baby checkups? Some pediatricians set aside special office hours or a separate area for the reception of newborns, which can be advantageous.

6. What are the doctor's feelings about breastfeeding and bottle-feeding? The answer to this question is crucial if you plan to nurse. A pediatrician's support and encouragement are very important for breastfeeding to be successful. Try to ascertain whether the doctor is only paying lip service to nursing or is sincerely supportive. If he says "breast is best," then follows up with "but many women find it inconvenient" or "many women don't have enough milk," he's given you a clue to his real feelings. By the same

token, if you plan to bottle-feed and the pediatrician is a La Leche League enthusiast, you're not going to feel very comfortable with him.

7. When does the doctor recommend introducing solid food? Experts generally agree that breast milk or formula provides all the nutrients most babies need for the first four to six months of life. If the doctor sets a rigid date for introducing solids rather than presenting a flexible, wait-and-see approach, he may not be right for you.
8. What are the doctor's feelings about circumcision? If religious reasons are not a factor, you should discuss the question of circumcision with the pediatrician. Many medical professionals are now advising that newborn males not be routinely circumcised.
9. What are the doctor's fees for well-baby checkups and for sick visits?
10. Does the doctor make house calls? This is rare, but some pediatricians still do.
11. If you are considering early discharge from the hospital, or if you plan to deliver at an alternative birth center or at home, you should discuss this with the pediatrician. Many alternative birth centers, in fact, require a consent form from your pediatrician.

Last, and probably least, look around the doctor's waiting and examining rooms. Since the pediatrician's office is a place where your child will have to feel comfortable, it helps if it is nicely decorated, with playthings and books for the children. If the waiting room is very crowded, ask the nurse or receptionist if there is a separate area for contagious children. Crowded pediatricians'

Preparing for Baby

offices are breeding grounds for illness. Of course, a one-time visit won't tell you whether the waiting room is always empty or crowded. There are seasonal illnesses, as well as seasonal visits because of a new school year or checkups for camp. You might casually say to the nurse or receptionist, "Is it always this peaceful?" or "Is it always this hectic? You must go crazy." Chances are her reply will be an honest, off-the-cuff one.

But don't let a waiting room fool you. There are some very terrific doctors with some boring waiting rooms. If the doctor appears perfect but his waiting room doesn't, take a chance on him.

If for some reason you become dissatisfied with the pediatrician you've chosen, don't hesitate to switch. Your personality and the doctor's may just not be a good match. If that's the case, changing doctors will help you both. You and your baby can easily get to know a new pediatrician. If you do decide to change, you'll have to let the doctor know so he can transfer the baby's records to your new pediatrician. You can sometimes accomplish this over the phone with the receptionist or nurse, but some doctors require a request in writing from the new doctor or from you in person.

6. Childbirth

As your due date approaches, you will be focusing more and more on the upcoming birth. You may even start dreaming about labor and delivery and what your new baby will be like. Many expectant parents take classes to become familiar with the events of childbirth and to learn techniques for managing labor and delivery. Practicing relaxation and breathing can give you a feeling of confidence and aid you when your baby's birthday arrives.

Preparing for Birth

"I was so eager to begin childbirth preparation classes that I called the local Lamaze chapter within days of having the pregnancy confirmed," recalls one mother. "I felt a little silly when they told me classes didn't begin until about eight weeks before my due date."

Although she may have jumped the gun a bit, this woman's enthusiastic attitude reflects one of the most important changes in the childbirth scene of the last 20 years.

Childbirth

Instead of approaching the due date with anxiety and a lack of information, expectant parents are preparing themselves by attending a variety of classes.

Of the 64,000 women who responded to a poll on labor and delivery experiences in the November 1981 issue of *Parents* Magazine, 85.5 percent said that they had attended childbirth preparation classes. Of those who took classes, 22.3 percent thought they were indispensable in controlling pain, 33 percent thought they were very helpful, and 33 percent thought they were helpful. The women responded similarly when asked how effective the techniques were in helping them to relax.

In addition, the presence of a prepared husband or other support person is not only allowed today but actually expected, for this person plays a crucial role in working with the expectant mother. The importance of providing support to a woman in labor cannot be overestimated. Among comparable groups of women, studies show that those who receive such support tend to manage their labors better and to need less medication than those who do not have support.

Many expectant parents are confused by the terms "prepared childbirth" and "natural childbirth." The terms are used almost interchangeably today, but they are really not the same. In making a distinction between them, it may be helpful to think of the first as designed to lead to the second.

Prepared childbirth, as noted above, means that the mother and her support person have taken a series of classes to prepare for the birth. Depending on where they are offered, who teaches them, and what the philosophy is, the classes could cover a wide range of topics from maternal nutrition and exercise to specific breathing and relaxation techniques for use during labor and delivery.

Natural childbirth, in its strictest sense, means that no medications are given during labor and delivery and that there are no interventions in the birth process. The term was originally used to contrast a prepared birth with what was the rule of the day earlier in this century—the routine use of medication for laboring women and the routine use of instruments to accomplish delivery. Today, a majority of women have had some degree of preparation, but natural childbirth remains, in people's minds and vocabularies, linked with other movements like natural foods.

There are several different methods of childbirth preparation. The first efforts to discover a way to make childbirth a less feared and painful event began almost simultaneously in Great Britain and the Soviet Union in the 1920s.

Grantly Dick-Read

A British obstetrician who is considered the father of prepared childbirth, Grantly Dick-Read developed a theory that a woman's fear of pain in labor can create tension, which in turn produces real pain. He called this the fear-tension-pain cycle. The spark for his pioneering work came when he attended the birth of a woman who was unafraid of birth pains and refused his offer of chloroform, the principal anesthetic used at the time. In what has become a legendary remark, the woman is reported to have said to Dick-Read after the birth, "It didn't hurt. It wasn't meant to, was it, doctor?"

Dick-Read offered classes to prepare his patients for labor and birth, describing the physiological process and teaching them relaxation and breathing techniques. He saw the value of a support person to assist the laboring woman, although most often that person was the doctor himself instead of the father of the baby. In 1933, his first book, called *Natural Childbirth*, was published in England. An expanded presentation of his method was published in the United States in 1944 under the title *Childbirth Without Fear*. Sales of the book and a number of lecture tours helped to advance his method in this country and throughout the world. Although many current classes of childbirth preparation include some of Dick-Read's concepts, there is no organization that teaches the Dick-Read method exclusively.

Fernand Lamaze

A different approach was taken by physicians in the Soviet Union who were experimenting with hypnosis and a method of pain control in labor that came to be known as psychoprophylaxis (literally, "mind prevention of disease"). It was based on the Pavlovian theory of conditioned response to a stimulus. In a famed experiment, Pavlov taught a dog, through conditioning, to salivate at the sound of a bell, because the ringing always preceded the arrival of food. The Russians felt that pregnant women could be similarly conditioned to respond to labor pains by relaxing rather than tensing their muscles, allowing the uterus to work efficiently.

A French obstetrician named Fernand Lamaze visited

the Soviet Union in the early 1950s and observed the technique, which by then had been mandated by the government as the officially endorsed method of childbirth. He was strongly impressed by its success and proceeded to adapt it for use with his own patients in France. He evolved a method of preparation that includes techniques to promote relaxation, a series of breathing patterns to match various levels of contractions in labor, and visual distraction—women concentrate on a specific object while breathing in an attempt to distract themselves from uterine activity. He also developed *effleurage*, a light massage of the mother's abdomen that serves as both a comfort measure and a distraction. All these techniques are practiced diligently with a support person in the weeks before the birth so that a conditioned response can be achieved.

An American woman named Marjorie Karmel, who had a birth by the Lamaze method in France, brought the method to the attention of the American public with her book *Thank You, Dr. Lamaze*, published in 1959. Along with a number of others, she founded the American Society for Psychoprophylaxis in Obstetrics (ASPO), which is the official Lamaze organization in the U.S. ASPO is headquartered in Virginia, but there are ASPO coordinators in each state as well as local groups.

ASPO has strict criteria for teacher certification; the process takes a year to a year and a half. Many Lamaze teachers are registered nurses as well.

Robert Bradley

At about the same time that the Lamaze method was being brought to the U.S., Robert Bradley, a young Denver obstetrician, was developing his own method of prepared childbirth derived from Dick-Read's principles. Bradley, who grew up on a farm, was intrigued by the difference between animal labor, which seemed peaceful and painless, and human labor, which was quite the opposite. Animals find a dark, quiet place in which to labor and give birth; they settle into a comfortable position and actually look and breathe as they do when asleep. His observations of animals led him to adapt their behavior to human experience. Moreover, he was the first to introduce husband coaches in labor; his method is also known as husband-coached childbirth, the title of his own book on the subject. The husband's loving support and assistance are considered essential to the laboring woman.

In the Bradley method, women are encouraged to assume their sleep position during labor and to relax and breathe abdominally. Although abdominal breathing is the only type taught aside from breath-holding for pushing in second stage labor, the Bradley series of classes is longer by several weeks than the Lamaze classes. They include exercises to improve comfort and flexibility during pregnancy, labor, and delivery; relaxation techniques; and classes on nutrition, among other subjects.

The American Academy of Husband-Coached Childbirth (AAHCC), the national organization of the Bradley method, was founded in California by Marjie and Jay Hathaway, whose fourth child was born with Dr. Bradley in attendance. Although the organization is strongest in Western states, its graduates are now teaching in most other areas of the U.S.

Like ASPO, the AAHCC has strict criteria for accrediting its teachers. Because the husband is considered to be so important, husbands and wives are encouraged to team teach. The Academy prefers that teachers experience a Bradley method birth themselves, although it may accept birth experiences in which other prepared childbirth techniques have been used. Bradley teachers are expected to achieve an unmedicated, spontaneous birth for 90 percent or more of the couples eligible for classes.

Lamaze and Bradley Compared

While both methods rely on relaxation and breathing techniques, the emphasis is really quite different. The central difference is that the Lamaze method teaches distraction from uterine activity through various patterns of chest breathing and by focusing on an external object, while the Bradley method teaches slow abdominal breathing and involvement in uterine activity by focusing inward.

Neither method promises painless childbirth but rather offers techniques to minimize and control whatever pain you feel. Bradley teachers do not believe in the use of medication unless it is necessary for serious discomfort. Lamaze teachers also attempt to minimize the use of pain relief but are less adamant about this point. In the Lamaze method, the husband's participation is important but not quite to the same degree as in the Bradley method. Bradley husbands are specifically taught to assist their wives during contractions by talking to them, helping them to relax, and serving as their advocates with the hospital staff.

Despite these variations, it is well to keep in mind that the differences discussed here may not be as pronounced in all Lamaze or Bradley classes. Each teacher is an individual and brings to her classes her own background, experience, and attitudes.

Sheila Kitzinger

A British anthropologist and childbirth educator, Sheila Kitzinger developed what she calls the psychosexual approach to birth, based partly on Dick-Read's methods. She also draws on psychoanalytic theory, social anthropology, and even on Stanislavsky's acting exercises. Stanislavsky used sensory memory and imaginary activity—for example, walking barefoot in sand—to explore the way the body functions. Kitzinger uses the same approach as an aid to relaxation.

Her principal relaxation technique is known as touch relaxation. In preparation for labor, a woman is taught to relax different parts of her body in response to her partner's touch, as if the partner were literally drawing tension out of her. The Kitzinger method teaches both chest and abdominal breathing, not as distractions but as another way of getting in tune with your body.

There is no organization that has officially adopted the Kitzinger method in the U.S., but many teachers incorporate some of her principles in their own classes. She has published several books describing the method.

Finding a Childbirth Preparation Class

From these descriptions and from conversations with expectant and new parents, you probably will have some idea of the method of childbirth preparation you prefer. The ASPO organization and the AAHCC should be able to direct you to someone in your area who teaches these specific methods. But many childbirth educators draw from more than one of the preparatory disciplines. The International Childbirth Education Association (ICEA), dedicated to family-centered maternity care, certifies teachers but espouses no particular method. ICEA members can direct you to an ICEA teacher in your community. Other organizations such as La Leche League and women's groups, and also your physician or nurse-midwife may have names to suggest too.

If you have the time and inclination, you may want to attend classes in more than one method. Says one mother who trained in both Bradley and Lamaze, "I wanted to have as many tools as possible available to me. And I found that I used everything I learned at different stages of labor and delivery."

Classes may be held in the teacher's home or move from one home to another of the couples in the group. They provide a great way to meet and establish a close relationship with other expectant parents in your area. Private classes are usually small and informal; an average of six to eight couples is best, because larger groups make individual instruction difficult. Private teachers may also be freer than those in hospitals to discuss your options

Childbirth

and priorities for the birth experience and can make suggestions for how best to achieve your goals.

With the increasing interest in family-centered maternity care, many hospitals offer childbirth preparation classes. There are pros and cons to taking a course at a hospital. The classes are usually larger than with a private teacher and are often taught by a hospital staff member. While a nurse on staff at the hospital will be able to give you useful insights into the working of the labor and delivery floor, she may sometimes be more inclined to teach you how to get along with hospital rules and routines than how to get what you want. But not all hospital classes are taught by staff members.

In addition to childbirth preparation, hospitals may offer other classes on a variety of topics, including breastfeeding, baby care, and cesarean birth. Some hospitals require parents to have taken their class on cesarean section in order to permit the father to attend a cesarean birth.

Whether or not you decide to take a hospital class, if you are planning on a hospital delivery, you should take a tour of the maternity floor to familiarize yourself with the environment. Most hospitals have daily or weekly tours that you can sign up for. The tours will also provide you with an opportunity to ask any questions you may have about hospital routines.

The Red Cross, YM-YWCAs, YM-YWHAs, and other community centers also may offer childbirth education classes. The Red Cross also offers a baby care class that many expectant parents find very helpful. "It made me feel I had some experience when the baby was born. I wasn't as scared to take care of him as I would have been without the course," says one new father.

Most childbirth classes, whether offered by a hospital or a private instructor, have reunions after all class members have had their babies. The reunions give you an opportunity to share your labor and delivery stories and to show off your baby.

The length of classes varies according to the method being taught and the instructor. Classes are generally two hours long, once a week for six to eight weeks. Although you may not need to sign up for a class as soon as your pregnancy is confirmed, it's a good idea to start checking early on, because in many communities the classes are filled early in advance.

The cost of childbirth classes varies according to the teacher, the size of the class, and your geographical location. Don't let the cost be a determining factor in the classes you choose, however. If the class you think you want is just too expensive, talk to the instructor. Teachers sometimes will adjust their fees for prospective students who can't afford them.

Postscript

Many of you may find it hard to be disciplined and to practice the relaxation and breathing techniques as often as you should. You may think that you've got it all down pat and don't need constant rehearsing, or you may feel bored with the repetition. But if you don't practice enough, you may find yourself without the resources you thought you'd have when the big day arrives. Asked what they would do differently if they had another baby, 32 percent of the respondents to the *Parents* poll replied, "Practice prepared childbirth techniques more." Of the eight possible answers, that response was checked most often. They're trying to tell you something.

Childbirth Medications

While every pregnant woman wonders how painful her labor will be, there is no way to know this in advance, just as there is no way to predict the length of labor. You've probably heard conflicting stories from friends. One may have spent 20 hours in intense labor while another may not have believed that she was in active labor because the contractions were so mild. The variety of stories only attests to labor's variability and unpredictability.

In the past, many childbirth educators were reluctant to discuss pain, as if by not acknowledging it and by emphasizing preparation methods they could prevent its onset. At most, they spoke only of discomfort. This reluctance actually worked against the purpose of prepared childbirth, because it meant that women might be caught off guard if they felt pain, then become tense and lose control. While preparation is essential in order to maintain control during labor and delivery, and for some women may truly provide a painless birth, the vast majority of laboring women will still experience some pain. How much pain and how well you tolerate it will depend on your preparation, the support you have, your own pain threshold, and the characteristics of your labor.

Childbirth preparation coupled with a supportive birth

environment can help reduce or eliminate the need for pain medication, barring complications. Although what Dr. Bradley calls the "knock 'em out, drag 'em out" approach was in vogue for many years, it is generally acknowledged today that the smallest effective amount of medication, and ideally no medication, is best for both baby and mother. All childbirth medications cross the placenta and affect the baby in various ways. They also have a variety of effects on the mother and on the course of labor. What effect a medication will have depends on the individual drug, the dosage, and when the drug is given.

Despite many of the drawbacks to medication, it does have a place in childbirth today. Unlike laboring women of the past, you can be prepared for childbirth and, if your labor becomes lengthy without relief, too intense, or if you have complications, you have medication to assist you. Medication does not promise a pain-free labor and delivery either. Because of the effects drugs can have on the mother, the baby, and labor, they can't be given from your first contraction through delivery of the placenta. Medications that offer the most complete pain relief in general can't be given until you are at least in active labor.

If you feel strongly about not receiving pain medication unless absolutely necessary, you should make this clear to your caregiver during your pregnancy. Ask about the medications that may be used, at what point they may be given, and what the benefits and drawbacks are to each one. Also ask what he recommends and why. Based on this discussion and your own reading on the subject, you should try to reach agreement on medication in advance. Ask to have this agreement noted in your medical record.

Pain relief falls into two general categories: analgesia,

which reduces the sensation of pain, and anesthesia, which eliminates all sensation, either in a particular area of the body or by inducing a state of unconsciousness.

Analgesia

While narcotics are the drugs that have a true analgesic effect, tranquilizers and sedatives are occasionally used in early labor. They do not actually relieve pain but can help a mother relax if she is unusually nervous and is having difficulty coping with contractions. They are generally not given during active labor because of their undesirable side effects. These include drowsiness, confusion, and dizziness in the mother, and poor muscle tone, lowered body temperature, and respiratory depression in the newborn.

The narcotic most commonly used during labor is Demerol®. Since it can prolong labor, it is generally not given until a mother is in active labor. Some women find that it helps them relax and that it takes the edge off the pain. Other women, however, find it ineffective for pain relief and say that it interferes with their ability to concentrate on their breathing and relaxation techniques. And side effects such as nausea and dizziness may compound a mother's discomfort, rather than relieve it. If a mother is given a large enough dose that she falls asleep between contractions, her coach will have to be very alert and awaken her as each contraction begins, so that she can get on top of it before it reaches its peak. If she isn't given time to get in control, the contractions will seem more painful. Narcotics can also have undesirable effects on the baby, particularly respiratory depression.

Timing is crucial when any drug is given during labor. After a drug has crossed the placenta and been carried to the baby's organs, it will be passed back to the mother to be excreted. This process takes time. If the baby is born before he has excreted the drug, he will have to metabolize it on his own. Because the newborn's liver and kidneys are immature, he cannot excrete the drug as quickly as necessary and the baby can be depressed. Although a caregiver will attempt to correctly estimate the time of delivery when he decides on the dosage and when and how to give a drug, the time of a baby's birth is difficult to accurately predict. The caregiver may think birth is four hours off—enough time for the fetus to excrete an injection of Demerol®, for instance—when the baby is actually born in two hours. If a baby is born with respiratory depression resulting from narcotics, he can be given an injection of Narcan®. This is a narcotic antagonistic, which means that it can help reverse the depressing effects of narcotics.

Anesthesia

There are three types of anesthesia: general, regional, and local. With the advent of prepared childbirth and our ever-expanding knowledge about drugs and their effects on the baby, general anesthesia has become a rarity in an uncomplicated vaginal delivery. General anesthesia, meaning a loss of consciousness, can be accomplished by IV injection or by inhalation of a gas. It is used today mostly for emergency situations, when a baby must be delivered immediately.

Childbirth

Regional anesthesia numbs the lower part of the body, and the two types most commonly used are the epidural and the spinal. Of the two, only the epidural can be started during the active phase of labor. With an epidural, a catheter is inserted through the lower back into the epidural space that surrounds the spinal column. The catheter remains in place and serves as a passageway through which an anesthetic can be administered as needed. In hospitals where skilled anesthesiologists are available, the epidural is considered the preferred regional anesthesia for women who must have pain relief, but it does have decided disadvantages. It can slow labor, making necessary the use of oxytocin and increasing the risk of cesarean section. In addition, the urge to push is often lost, and this may lead to a forceps delivery. If a mother has practiced her pushing exercises well and is coached and supported, she may be able to push the baby out even with an epidural, but it takes more time. Other risks include a drop in maternal blood pressure, which will decrease the amount of oxygen reaching the baby, and postpartum backache. When time permits, an epidural is often used for a cesarean section. It allows the mother to be awake and to be with her baby immediately after birth. In many hospitals, prepared fathers are permitted to attend cesarean deliveries performed under regional anesthesia.

The spinal is also commonly used for a cesarean section. When it is used for a vaginal delivery, it can only be administered during second stage labor. This is the pushing stage, which many women find the most exhilarating part of the entire birth experience. Because it is given so late, a spinal is not helpful for most of the time a mother may need pain relief. She will lose the urge to push, and forceps will usually be required to deliver the baby. A spinal is administered with a single injection of anesthetic into the lower back. The most common side effect is the notorious spinal headache. The saddle block is a modified spinal that anesthetizes only the portion of the body that would touch a saddle if you were riding. It is commonly used during second stage labor for a forceps delivery.

Another type of regional anesthesia is the caudal. It is used less frequently today than in the past and has been mostly replaced by the epidural. With a caudal, an anesthetic is administered through a needle inserted at the base of the spinal column near the rectum. This method requires larger doses of anesthetic than an epidural, and there is the additional risk of puncturing the baby's head.

Local anesthesia numbs only a limited area of the body, and there are three types: the paracervical, pudendal, and perineal blocks.

Of the three, only the paracervical block is administered during first stage labor. With this method, an anesthetic is injected at regular intervals into the tissues surrounding the cervix. This numbs the area and helps reduce the pain of contractions. With a paracervical, the anesthetic quickly crosses the placenta and enters the baby's bloodstream, which can result in a drop in the baby's heart rate. Another risk is that a paracervical can prolong labor.

The perineal block is used only for an episiotomy and its repair. With a perineal, an anesthetic is injected just under the skin of the perineum—the area between the vagina and the anus.

The pudendal is used to numb the vagina for delivery,

and also to perform and repair an episiotomy. Some physicians also use it for a low forceps delivery. With a pudendal, an anesthetic is injected into both sides of the vagina.

Whether or not you use pain medication during labor and delivery will depend on many factors—the quality of your labor, its length, your ability to manage with prepared childbirth techniques, the support of those around you, and any complicating factors that may arise. Knowing what choices you have, and what the advantages and disadvantages are to each type of medication, will help you weigh the risks and make the best decision along with your caregiver.

Labor and Delivery

"I remember so clearly my reaction to losing my mucous plug two and a half weeks before my due date," laughs one mother of a six-month-old. "My heart started beating real fast, I had goose bumps, and, as I came out of the bathroom to tell my husband, all I could say was, 'I'm not ready, I'm not ready.' We looked at each other in disbelief, and my husband echoed me: 'I'm not ready either!'"

Every pregnant woman approaches labor and delivery with a mixture of excitement and fear. The day you've spent nine long months waiting for has finally arrived but, tired as you are of your cumbersome body, you're not quite sure you're ready to end the intimacy of carrying your child inside you. You're not sure you're ready, either, for the unknown of labor and delivery. But as labor truly gets under way, the feelings of unreadiness will fade, and you will look forward with excitement and joy to greeting your new baby.

Prelabor

Your body will begin preparing for labor several weeks before labor actually begins. If this is a first pregnancy, your baby may "drop" or become engaged at about the 36th week. This is called lightening, and it means that the baby's head or presenting part has descended into the pelvis. You can often tell when this has happened because you will be breathing easier, have less heartburn, and may feel fewer kicks right up against your ribs. Your profile will also change, and the belly bulge will be lower. In a second or subsequent pregnancy, lightening usually doesn't take place until after labor has begun.

During the eighth or ninth month, you will probably experience Braxton Hicks contractions. These contractions occur periodically throughout pregnancy but become stronger and more frequent in the final weeks. They are usually painless, but not always. Braxton Hicks contractions do not cause the cervix to dilate or open and so are signs of false labor. They occur irregularly and last for varying lengths of time. Braxton Hicks contractions usually subside if you relax or change your activity, while true labor contractions will continue no matter what you do. False labor can be annoying because you keep getting geared up for the big event. Its only real advantage, if you can call it that, is that you get a chance to practice

Childbirth

your prepared childbirth techniques with something resembling a real contraction. The practice can help you feel more confident of your ability to handle real labor contractions.

In the hours or days before labor begins, some women experience a burst of energy. They may feel like cleaning the whole house, running a dozen errands, or setting up the baby's room. This burst of energy is sometimes called the nesting instinct and is a mother's instinctual desire to make everything ready for her baby's arrival. If you do feel this burst of energy, it's important not to give in to it completely. If your instinct is accurate and labor will begin soon, it's best to conserve your energy for the work that lies ahead. If your instinct was premature and labor doesn't begin, you will have the time to do the cleaning or errands, and you'll be able to accomplish them more gradually and with less of a drain on your system.

Loss of the mucous plug, which keeps the cervical opening sealed during pregnancy, is often a sign that labor is imminent. The mucus is usually tinged with blood, and release of the plug is sometimes called a "pink show" or a "bloody show." Losing the plug, however, does not mean that labor will begin in a matter of hours. You could go into labor that quickly, but it may also be several days or even one or two weeks before labor begins. Some women pass the mucous plug without even noticing, or it may be discharged during labor.

What Is Labor?

The work of labor contractions is to completely efface and dilate the cervix—that is, to thin and open it. Effacement is measured in terms of percentages. When the cervix is 100 percent effaced, it is paper thin. Partial effacement often occurs during the last weeks of pregnancy. You may enter labor 25 or 50 or 80 percent effaced, for example. Dilation is measured in terms of centimeters. A fully dilated cervix is 10 centimeters—about 4 inches—and wide enough to allow for passage of the baby's head. You may also be slightly dilated when labor begins. First-time mothers, however, usually aren't as dilated as mothers having a second or subsequent baby.

Signs of True Labor

The onset of labor will be evident in one of two ways: you will experience contractions that are regular and increase in frequency and intensity as time passes, or your membranes or bag of waters will rupture.

Only about 10 percent of women experience spontaneous rupture of the membranes before labor begins. For most women, the membranes rupture at some point during labor. If the membranes do rupture ahead of time and the pregnancy is near term, chances are that labor will begin within 24 hours.

You should call your physician or nurse-midwife immediately if your membranes rupture before labor starts.

Childbirth

Some caregivers want a mother to be in the hospital or birth center as soon as the membranes have broken. Other caregivers, however, believe that in most cases, it's best for the mother to remain at home and active to help bring on contractions naturally. If you are asked to go to the hospital before labor begins, talk to your caregiver about being allowed mobility. If you don't ask, you will most likely be confined to bed upon admittance. Sitting or lying quietly in bed will not help labor to start. In addition, boredom and discouragement can be mentally wearing. "My membranes were leaking the night before and I still hadn't gone into labor the next morning, so my doctor admitted me to the hospital," recalls one mother. "I was confined to bed in the admitting labor room. My husband and I watched at least four other women being admitted in early labor. They sat with their coaches doing *effluerage* and breathing across from me, were switched to private rooms as their labor became active, and probably were all delivered before I had my first contraction. When I was finally induced late that afternoon, my heart wasn't in it anymore. I was unhappy, discouraged, and cranky." If contractions haven't begun in a certain amount of time, labor will probably be induced. Some physicians wait 12 hours; others, 24.

If your membranes rupture all at once, there will be no mistaking what has happened. You might hear a pop as the membranes break, and you will feel a good deal of warm, clear liquid gush out of your vagina. Ruptured membranes are painless, but it is certainly a wet experience. Many women concerned about membranes rupturing put a waterproof covering over their mattresses to protect their beds in case their waters break at night. (One

Lamaze teacher jokingly tells husbands to wear raincoats to bed in the last couple of weeks of pregnancy.) Here was one mother's plan in case her membranes ruptured at a grocery store: "I was very concerned about my membranes rupturing in public," she explains. "Actually, I was obsessed by the idea for some reason, even though everyone kept telling me how unlikely it was to happen. So when I was grocery shopping I first went to the juice aisle and put a half gallon of apple juice in my shopping cart. I figured if my membranes ruptured, I'd just drop the bottle of juice on the floor and pretend that was why the floor was wet."

Some women's waters only leak. This can be harder to identify, since you may be leaking small amounts of urine when you are near term because of the enlarged uterus pressing against the bladder. If you suspect a leak but aren't sure, call your caregiver. She can easily detect the presence of amniotic fluid by using a piece of yellow nitrazine paper. Amniotic fluid is very alkaline and will turn the yellow paper blue. If your membranes rupture or leak, you should not take a bath, use a tampon, or have sexual intercourse.

In the past, it was believed that labor would be harder and longer if the membranes ruptured in advance because the birth canal would be dry instead of wet. This simply is not true. Amniotic fluid is continually manufactured at a rate of about ¾ cup per hour until the baby is born. So if your membranes rupture early, not only will you not be dry, you will be wetter, since you will be leaking fluid continually. (This can be uncomfortable—it's like being in a wet diaper all day.) Wearing a sanitary pad and changing it frequently will help, but you'll still be damp.

Childbirth

Most often, membranes rupture spontaneously near the end of first stage labor, when the cervix is almost fully dilated. Very rarely, a baby will be born with unruptured membranes (this is called a caul). When this happens, the caregiver will immediately rupture the membranes so that the baby can begin breathing without inhaling amniotic fluid.

The majority of women go into labor with contractions that have some regularity, although the contractions are not always easily identifiable. Many women do not suspect that the achy feelings in their backs or the menstruallike cramps that come and go are actually early contractions. It may take a while for it to occur to you that these could be contractions. Often, if you time these sensations, you will find that they occur at set intervals and last for a set amount of time. As labor progresses, the contractions will usually become stronger, longer, and closer together.

Since every woman's labor is different, every woman's labor will begin differently as well. Throughout this chapter, we will discuss the events of labor in terms of generalities—the way things often happen—then try to give you an idea of the variations that can occur. Many mothers interviewed for this book have stressed that the most important advice to give women about labor is that it does not proceed according to a pat schedule or plan, and that they should expect the unexpected. If you know that in advance, you won't become so worried or discouraged by deviations from what you understand to be "normal."

Labor is divided into three stages. The first stage, which is the longest, covers the time from the onset of labor to full dilation of the cervix. This stage is itself divided into three phases: latent (dilation from 0 to 3 centimeters), active (dilation from 4 to 7 centimeters), and transition (dilation from 8 to 10 centimeters). The second stage of labor is the expulsion stage, when you push the baby down the birth canal and into the world. The third stage is the separation and delivery of the placenta.

First Stage Labor

As we've seen, labor can begin quietly, with contractions sort of sneaking up on you. It can also begin stormily, with contractions that are very intense. Or it can begin with any variation in between. If early or latent labor occurs at night, you may actually sleep through this phase and be awakened by contractions that are strong and regular. You may not even recognize the latent phase, depending on the character of your particular labor.

During the latent phase, the cervix effaces 100 percent and dilates to 3 centimeters. The contractions are usually mild, and relatively short and far apart. You and your coach should time the contractions so that you know how long they're lasting and how far apart they are, and then forget about timing for a while. You'll be able to tell when the character of the contractions is changing or when they are coming more frequently. When you think there's been a change, you can time them again. Many couples make the mistake of getting overinvolved with timing contractions. The coach is so busy looking at his stopwatch or the second hand on his clock and writing everything down that he forgets to pay attention to his wife—or to himself. So much concentration on timing—especially if the contractions are frequent—can be unnecessarily wearing. Some husbands are so overcome with nervousness and excitement that timing contractions and writing serve as a crutch—it defines the activity and distracts them from the reality of the situation. If you feel your coach is paying more attention to fiddling with the watch and paper than he is to you, make sure you let him know—and the earlier in labor the better. Some husbands seem to know just what to do when labor begins, and others need some coaching themselves. Since you will be counting on his support more and more as labor intensifies, you should talk out what you feel and need at the beginning.

What to Take to the Hospital

You should pack two separate bags if you are going to deliver in a hospital. One should be a bag with things you'll want to have during labor; the other is the suitcase with things you'll need during your hospital stay. Here are some suggestions for both:

Labor Bag

1. Wash cloths
2. Tennis balls for back pressure during back labor
3. A pair of socks if you get cold feet (literally, not figuratively!)
4. A lip balm for dry lips
5. Books, cards, lap games, or other distractions for early labor
6. Phone numbers of the people you'll want to call right after the birth
7. Lollipops—especially sour flavors—to suck on between contractions. Sour ones will ease nausea better than sweet flavors. Lollipops are better than hard candy because of the stick. You can hold it, keep it dipped in cold water during contractions, and don't have to worry about swallowing it by mistake
8. Talcum powder for *effluerage* and back rubs
9. A photograph or picture to concentrate on if you want a focal point
10. Camera and film
11. Paper and pen for timing contractions or keeping a journal of your labor and birth experience

228 PARENTS℠ BOOK OF PREGNANCY AND BIRTH

12. A watch or stopwatch
13. Contact lens case and contact solution, if you wear lenses, and a pair of glasses
14. Snack or thermos of coffee for coach

Suitcase

1. A couple of nightgowns, and if you plan to nurse, be sure they allow easy access to the breasts. You may prefer hospital gowns, since they're short. You can even wear one opening in front instead of in back
2. Nursing bras
3. Toothpaste, toothbrush
4. Slippers
5. Bathrobe
6. Shampoo, soap, deodorant, and other toiletries
7. Blowdryer
8. Watch or clock
9. Books
10. Announcements, if you have them in advance
11. Sanitary belt and pads. The hospital will probably provide a belt and will definitely give you thick pads, but you may prefer your own
12. Book on breastfeeding
13. Address book with phone numbers
14. Going-home clothes. These should either be maternity clothes or some large, comfortable clothes, because you won't be back to your pre-pregnant size quite yet. You don't necessarily have to pack these if you'll be staying at least overnight. Your husband or friends can always bring them later
15. Baby's going-home clothes. You don't necessarily have to pack these either, but you may want to. You'll need an undershirt and whatever other clothing is suitable for the time of year, and probably a hat and blanket.

During the latent phase, you should try to get as much rest as possible, especially if it occurs at night. With all the excitement of labor beginning, though, that may be difficult. Your husband should rest as well. Coaching is labor, too, and the more rested your husband is, the better he'll be able to help you. In between resting, your husband (and you, if you feel like it) can get things together if you

Childbirth

haven't already. He can pack your suitcase, or add the last-minute items if it's already packed, and fix himself a sandwich to take to the hospital or birth center. Food for the coach is very important. Coaches use up a lot of energy and need food to keep themselves going. You're probably not going to want to let your husband out of your sight once you arrive at the birth setting. Your husband might also want to do some last-minute dishes and bed-making, but straightening up should be secondary to resting and coaching. If he (or you) has the time and inclination to do it, fine. If not, just forget about it.

The latent phase of labor can last as long as 20 hours for a first-time mother and up to 14 hours for a woman giving birth for a second or subsequent time. Generally, however, it doesn't last this long. It's good to keep in mind that you probably won't be in much discomfort during the latent phase, even if it is long.

As you enter the active phase of labor, the contractions will pick up in intensity and become more defined. Each woman experiences contractions differently, but they are often described as wavelike because the contraction builds in intensity to a peak, then gradually subsides, like a wave cresting and breaking on the shore. The contraction can feel like a clamping down, a squeezing back pain, but rarely as a sharp pain like banging your elbow. Although the pain of a contraction is a very specific feeling for the woman experiencing it, most women find it difficult to describe and even more difficult to recall shortly after delivery.

During the active phase of labor, the cervix dilates from 4 to 7 centimeters. Contractions not only become more intense but longer and closer together. A very small percentage of women do not experience regular contractions or ones that get progressively closer together. "I was under the impression that once labor got started I would just get going. But for twenty-four hours I had contractions six then seven then eight minutes apart, then five minutes apart. Then they'd go back to six to seven or eight," says one new mother. "It was frustrating to labor so long without making progress. I expected labor to be horribly painful, but I was psyched. I was ready for it, but it just wasn't giving me a chance."

Even if your contractions seem to be progressing nicely, becoming stronger and closer together, you can't predict that you are advancing the 1 centimeter an hour that is the average. Actually, averages are pretty meaningless unless the labor is a prolonged one. Some women have strong, frequent contractions for hours and, when examined, find they haven't even progressed from 1 to 2 centimeters. Others have milder contractions at greater intervals and presume they're only 3 centimeters dilated when, in fact, they're 5 or 6. If you don't expect to dilate in a particular amount of time, you won't be disappointed if it seems to take you a long time to dilate from centimeter to centimeter. That's not to say you should expect a lengthy labor; it's just that the rhythm of each labor is different. You could spend a long time in the latent phase or in the active phase or even in transition (although this is more rare). You could progress rapidly from 1 to 5 centimeters and then get hung up. Or you could progress slowly from 1 to 5 and then proceed to full dilation with great speed. Or you might just dilate from centimeter to centimeter on a very regular and steady basis.

At some point either in the latent or active phase of

Childbirth

labor, you may feel overwhelmed by the inevitability of birth and the lack of control you have over it. There are few situations in life like this where your body will work on its own whether you want it to or not, despite how you feel. This lack of control has probably been an issue for you during pregnancy, and it logically continues now.

When to Call the Caregiver During your last month of pregnancy, your physician or nurse-midwife should explain when to call her once labor starts. Some caregivers want to be notified if a mother has any contractions, just to be kept informed. Others specify how far apart contractions should be before a mother calls. If your caregiver has examined you a few days before labor starts, he will know whether your cervix has begun to efface and dilate, and if so, how much. This information, together with the frequency and length of your contractions when you call, will help him determine when you should leave for the hospital or birth center. Many professionals advise that a first-time mother remain at home until contractions are about 5 to 8 minutes apart. A mother who is giving birth for a second or subsequent time may be asked to come in earlier, since her labor is likely to be quicker. Of course, how soon you leave depends on other factors too, including how far you live from the hospital or birth center and whether there is any indication that your labor will be speedier than most. In addition, if some potential problem is suspected, your caregiver may want you to arrive at the hospital early in labor.

The longer you can labor at home, the more relaxed and comfortable you will be. At home you can walk around, lie down, sit, squat, or assume any position you want. Mobility during first stage labor is crucial not only to your comfort but also to good progress in labor, because it encourages stronger and more efficient contractions. Women who walk around during labor generally have shorter labors than women who don't. Your husband may also be more relaxed at home and may be able to grab a bite to eat between helping you with contractions. Women are often hypersensitive to odors when they are in labor, and their coaches should be aware of this. One woman recalls that any smell of food was nauseating to her. "At one point," she says, "I had to put a towel under our apartment door because of cooking smells from other apartments!" An additional advantage to remaining home as long as possible is that friends or relatives can join you and help you and your coach. Of course, some couples prefer to labor alone, but many find the presence of another person very comforting, especially if it's a woman who has gone through labor. She can help make you comfortable by massaging your legs or back while your coach breathes with you or puts cold cloths on your face, and she can relieve the coach so he can get something to eat or rest. One mother who had a friend with her says, "It was wonderful having her there. She timed contractions, rubbed my back, and let my husband take a nap. It gave me a lift to have the two of them encouraging me, saying that I was doing well. My husband would say later that the most important thing during labor was having our friend there to lend support. It's exhausting work to be the coach, especially if you don't have everything ready and it has to be done between contractions."

Some couples, of course, do not feel comfortable or at ease until they have arrived at the hospital or birth center. They may be too concerned about getting there

Childbirth

in time, or they may simply feel more protected in the professional environment. If that's the case, don't linger at home. The best place for you to be is where you feel most relaxed and comfortable.

Arriving at the Birth Setting When you arrive at the hospital or birth center, you will be asked about your labor—when it began, how far apart the contractions are and how long they are lasting, whether your membranes ruptured, whether you had a bloody show. You will also be given an internal examination to determine how effaced and dilated you are. If you are indeed in progressive labor, you will be formally admitted. What happens next depends on where you are giving birth and what arrangements you worked out with your caregiver ahead of time. As we discussed in part one, there are a number of routine admitting procedures that are associated with a hospital birth, including pubic shaves, enemas, and IVs. While they may not be as routine as they once were, they are still commonly done. If you want to avoid these procedures, you should discuss it with your physician early in pregnancy, then reconfirm what was agreed upon during one of your final prenatal visits. At an alternative birth center, there are no routine shaves, enemas, or IVs.

Once you are settled in the labor or birthing room, you will be examined periodically to determine how effaced and dilated you are, and how far the baby's head or presenting part has descended into the pelvis. Usually, internal examinations are kept to a minimum, especially if the membranes have ruptured, since there is some risk of infection once this has happened. Internal exams are uncomfortable—and can be extremely painful, especially when they are done during contractions. You should ask your caregiver to do the exams between contractions, which is a little more tolerable. Although the exams may hurt, when you find that you have progressed, your spirits will soar. (The opposite can also be true, of course. It's very discouraging to labor long and hard, and find that dilation isn't progressing or is going very slowly.) In fact, many women find that if their mood and strength are failing, an examination showing progress can be more of a shot in the arm than a real shot of medication.

It's at some point in the active phase of labor that you may feel like requesting medication—or that medication will be offered to you. Whether or not you ask for or receive medication will depend entirely on the character of your labor and on your own pain threshold. It is often suggested that you try to wait 30 minutes to an hour after you first feel like asking for medication or after it's first offered. When the time is up, you can reevaluate how you feel and can also ask for an internal exam. Sometimes a great deal of progress is unexpectedly made in a very short period of time, and the medication that seemed so enticing is simply no longer necessary.

There are many things that you can do to help keep yourself comfortable during the active phase of labor, and since you may be concentrating very hard on dealing with contractions, your coach should keep these foremost in mind. Walk around if you feel like it. You can always stop to lean against your coach, a wall, or to drape yourself over a chair when a contraction comes. If you don't feel like walking, position changes in bed can be helpful as well. If you're lying on your side, switch to a semisitting position, with pillows under your knees and elbows so that all your joints are relaxed. Leg and arm massages

Childbirth

can sometimes feel great in between or even during contractions. Cold compresses on your forehead or having your face and neck wiped with a cold cloth will also feel good. If you are giving birth at an alternative birth center, you will probably be allowed to have water, juice, tea, or broth during labor. Some hospitals also allow sips of liquid, but many only allow ice chips. A few hospitals don't even permit ice chips, in which case sucking on or wiping your lips with a cold, wet washcloth can be soothing.

You may not notice that your bladder is full because of the contractions and the feeling of pressure that you have in the pelvic area, so be sure to empty your bladder about once an hour. If your bladder is empty, you'll feel more comfortable and your labor may progress better. If you're allowed to go to the bathroom, do so. If you're attached to an IV or fetal monitor, or not allowed out of bed, ask the nurse for a bedpan. One woman remembers finding the bedpan awkward and inhibiting. "But the nurse was smart," she says. "When she saw I was having trouble, she turned on the water faucet in the room. The sound of water running triggered my bladder, and I was able to urinate."

During the active phase of labor, you may go through mood changes as well as physical changes as the contractions become stronger and closer together. While you may have talked excitedly and animatedly during the latent phase and even during the beginning of the active phase, the contractions are going to demand more and more concentration from you, and you may find that you retreat from those around you. Although many women feel that they are aware of everything during their labors, they discover that when they try to recall the events, much of what happened is a blur. Make sure that you let your coach know what you want. If you like being talked to and soothed in between or during contractions, tell him. When your needs change, let him know. You'll wish sometimes that your coach could divine what you want, but it's unrealistic to expect him to.

When you enter transition, you are nearing the end of first stage labor. During this final phase, the cervix dilates from 8 centimeters to 10. Transition is the hardest and most challenging phase of first stage labor, but it is also the shortest. There are many signs and symptoms of transition, and while few women experience all of them, most women experience some. They include the following:

1. An increase in the intensity and length of contractions, with less time to rest in between. The contractions can be very intense, may have more than one peak, and can last up to 1½ to 2 minutes, with only a very short interval between them. There will almost always be some time between contractions, but it may be so short as to be imperceptible to you.
2. You may become nauseous or vomit.
3. Your legs may tremble or shake, and you might get leg cramps.
4. You may experience temperature changes—you may feel very hot, then very cold.
5. There may be a feeling of intense pressure in your rectum as the baby descends, and you may be convinced that you have to have a bowel movement.
6. You may feel a strong urge to push. If you do, be sure to resist it and to call a nurse or your caregiver im-

Childbirth

mediately. The urge to push usually accompanies full dilation, but it can come earlier. You should not push until you are fully dilated. If you push too soon, the cervix may swell or even tear.
7. You may feel that you can't go on any longer. A common request of women in transition is to go home and come back and finish tomorrow. You may feel panicky, lose control, and become very irritable. Many women suddenly don't want to be touched by their coaches, even when touching was helpful before, and snap at anything their coaches say.

If you exhibit any of these signs, it is a signal to your coach that you may be in transition. Once he and you realize this, you will feel much better, as the birth of your baby is very near.

You will need all the support and encouragement you can get at this time. At some point during transition, you may suddenly feel that you can't go on without medication. While it may be tempting to ask for an anesthetic, transition is usually so short that it's a shame to be anesthetized now and to be numbed for the birth. Transition usually lasts about 30 minutes, but can be as short as one or two contractions or as long as two hours. For many women, just knowing that they're in transition allows them to get through it. It's the thought that labor is going to get even worse that makes women ask for pain relief. If you're in transition, the pain is not going to get worse. The worst, in fact, is just about over.

Second Stage Labor

Once you are fully dilated and have been given the go-ahead to push, your outlook will most likely change drastically. Pushing is the part of labor that requires you to be active, rather than passive. Many women find pushing a tremendous relief, especially if the urge to push is strong and they feel they are working in concert with their bodies. Everyone agrees that pushing is the hardest work they've ever done, and most of the women interviewed for this book felt that they hadn't fully realized the extent of the effort required. Some women find that pushing is painful, not painless, as it is generally described. "I was surprised how much it hurt during the final pushing stage," says one new mother. "I'd read so much about what a release it is. But for me it hurt just about as much as anything else that day." A small percentage of women never feel the urge to push or don't feel it as the tremendous force that the majority do. For these women, pushing can be more difficult, simply because they have to be coached to do something they don't feel. If you've received regional anesthesia, you probably won't feel the urge to push either.

First-time mothers generally spend longer pushing their babies out than mothers having a second or subsequent baby, but how long it takes depends on your contractions, the baby's size and position, and your own size as well. It's not unusual for a first-time mother to push for two hours, although most women push for a much shorter time.

Childbirth

The contractions that accompany second stage labor are usually further apart than the contractions of transition. It often takes at least a few contractions to get the hang of pushing, and your caregiver and coach will help you by giving you verbal cues: "Okay, take a deep breath, breathe out, breathe in, hold it and push!" It's very important as you push to keep your perineal area relaxed. Keeping your jaw slack while pushing usually helps relax the perineal area—it's like the two are held together with the same string. (You know how your mouth usually opens while you're putting on mascara, despite your efforts to keep it closed? It's the same idea.) You'll probably do several pushes with each contraction. When progress is being made, those who attend your delivery become like a cheerleading squad, urging you on and giving you confidence in your ability.

Your position during second stage labor can either be comfortable and assist your pushing efforts or uncomfortable and actually hamper progress. The lithotomy position, in which you lie flat on your back, is the most uncomfortable and the least effective. It diminishes the amount of effort you can exert, and works against the force of gravity. Also, when you lie flat on your back, the baby's weight compresses major blood vessels, which impedes your circulation and the baby's. Squatting is by far the most effective position for second stage labor. There is no adverse effect on circulation, and the force of gravity is used to its utmost. Many women prefer to sit up with their backs supported. The advantages of this position are similar to those for squatting. When you're in a sitting position, you can bend your knees and pull your legs up toward your body as you push. This will add force to the pushing movements. Some women feel most comfortable lying on their side. This position does not hinder circulation or the strength of contractions. Your top leg, however, will have to be raised when you push. You can do this yourself, but it may be very tiring. Your coach or a nurse can do it for you, or if you are on a delivery table, your leg can be placed on one of the stirrups.

If you are giving birth in a hospital with traditional labor-delivery facilities, you will be moved from the labor to the delivery room when the baby's birth seems imminent. The move is often made once the baby's head has crowned, which means that the top of the head can be seen at the vaginal opening. In a second or subsequent labor, the transfer may be made sooner, since delivery can be quite speedy. If you are giving birth in a hospital birthing room or at an alternative birth center, you will labor and deliver in the same room and bed, and you have more freedom to assume a birth position you find most comfortable. There are many advantages to remaining in the same place for labor and delivery. The greatest is that you don't have to be moved just when you are experiencing some of the most intense feelings of labor. Some physicians and hospitals allow mothers who are having prepared, uncomplicated births to deliver in the labor room. If you will be having a hospital birth and the hospital does not have a birthing room, this is something that you may want to discuss with your physician ahead of time. Until quite recently, the traditional birth position was the lithotomy or flat-on-the-back position, with legs far apart and feet in stirrups. It is the least effective position for a prepared, uncomplicated birth because it works

Childbirth

against the force of gravity. Progressive physicians and hospitals do not encourage this position for mothers who are actively participating in birth. Most modern delivery tables can be adjusted so that the mother can be in a semisitting position rather than on her back. If the delivery table cannot be adjusted, a backrest may be supplied. In this position, the mother can keep her knees bent and her feet flat on the delivery table rather than in stirrups. If you will be giving birth in a hospital delivery room, you should discuss birth positions with your physician early in pregnancy. While the lithotomy position may be necessary in certain situations, such as forceps delivery, it is inappropriate for prepared, uncomplicated births.

Whether you are in a birthing room or a delivery room, excitement will intensify as more and more of the baby's head or presenting part becomes visible. During this time, your caregiver will assess the need for an episiotomy, an incision made between the vagina and anus to enlarge the vaginal opening (see page 242). When the baby's head is about to be born, you will be instructed to stop pushing and to pant so that the head can be eased out. In most cases, the baby's face will be facing down but will spontaneously turn to the right or the left so that the head is aligned with the rest of the body. Once the head is born, your caregiver will probably use a small syringe to suction mucus from the baby's mouth. The shoulders are then delivered, first the top one, then the bottom. After this, the rest of the body slips out quickly and easily. As the body is being delivered, your caregiver may again suction the baby's mouth in preparation for the baby's first full breath.

> ### Is an Episiotomy Necessary?
>
> *The routine use of episiotomy is currently the subject of much debate. It's been estimated that 80 to 90 percent of women giving birth for the first time have episiotomies, together with about 50 percent of women giving birth for a second or subsequent time. Several reasons are generally cited for routine episiotomy: it helps guard against possible tearing; it provides a clean cut which is easier to repair than a laceration; it eases delivery of the baby's head, helping to protect it from possible compression; and it helps prevent possible sexual and gynecological problems that may result from tearing or overstretching. Those who question routine episiotomy point out that there is currently no scientific evidence to prove these contentions. They also note that a tear is not automatically going to result. A woman who has taken prepared childbirth classes and who is actively participating in birth can better control the urge to push and can ease the baby out slowly and carefully, minimizing the possibility of tearing. There are also problems associated with episiotomy, including possible infection and painful intercourse because of improper healing or suturing. While the routine use of episiotomy is being questioned, you should be aware that there are situations in which an episiotomy is necessary, including forceps delivery and a birth in which the baby's head is too large for the vaginal opening. Also, if it is evident that a bad tear will occur, an episiotomy is obviously preferable. You should discuss your caregiver's views about episiotomy well before the birth, and you should also make your own preferences known. Whether or not an episiotomy is necessary is a medical judgment that can only be made at the time of delivery, and the decision will ultimately rest with the caregiver. Ideally, you should have confidence in his judgment and he should have respect for your preferences.*

The birth is such an emotional event, especially after the hard work of labor, that the relief can be overwhelming. Tears of joy and release are common for both mothers and fathers, and for most, the thrill of seeing the baby erases the hours of pain and uncertainty that preceded it. One mother who during transition remembers telling her husband that one child was going to be just fine, thank

Childbirth

you, also remembers turning to her husband just after the birth and saying, "Oh, let's do this again, honey!"

When the baby is given to you will depend on where you are giving birth and what arrangements you made with your caregiver ahead of time. In a more traditional hospital birth, the baby is usually checked first, cleaned up a bit, then wrapped in a blanket and given to the mother to hold. In a family-centered environment, the baby is usually laid tummy-down on the mother's abdomen immediately after birth, and the umbilical cord may not be cut until it stops pulsating. Skin-to-skin contact is thought to enhance the bonding process, and delaying cutting the cord lets the baby get oxygen through both the cord and lungs, and may help ease his adjustment from womb to world. If you want to hold your baby right after birth and to have skin-to-skin contact, you should discuss this with your physician ahead of time. And if you want to nurse on the delivery table, you should let him know. While not all babies are interested in nursing right away, the skin contact will be soothing to your baby and to you, and even a slight nuzzling of your nipple will help the uterus contract and hasten delivery of the placenta. You should also ask if prophylactic eye drops can be delayed until you and your husband have had a chance to hold and interact with your newborn. These drops protect the baby's eyes in case the mother has gonorrhea and are required by law in most states. The drops, however, blur the baby's vision, which interferes with the eye-to-eye contact that many researchers believe enhances the bonding process.

Your baby's condition will be assessed at one minute and again at five minutes after birth according to an evaluation scale developed by Dr. Virginia Apgar. The Apgar score is assigned when your baby has been checked on five physical functions: heart rate, respiration, muscle tone, reflexes, and skin color. He will receive 0 to 2 points for each. Most babies score 7 or above, and the scores are usually higher on the second evaluation than on the first. Babies with scores below 7 may need assistance with breathing and will be carefully watched in the hours immediately following birth.

Third Stage Labor

To you, childbirth may be over once your baby is born, but the birth process is not completed until the placenta has been delivered and examined. Your uterus will continue to contract after the baby's birth, although you may not always be aware of the contractions. The continued contractions help the placenta separate from the uterine wall. When it has fully detached, your caregiver will ask you to give a good push or two to deliver it. He may also put a small amount of traction on the umbilical cord to speed the delivery. Delivery of the placenta is usually painless or only slightly uncomfortable. The placenta will probably be larger than you imagined and has a rough side, which was lying against the uterine wall, and a smooth, shiny side, which was lying toward the baby. If you're interested, ask to see the placenta. It's an amazing organ.

The placenta will be carefully examined to ensure that pieces of it have not been left inside you. Any piece of placenta that remains in the uterus can cause postpartum hemorrhage. Some doctors routinely examine the inside of the uterus manually after the placenta is delivered to make sure that no pieces were left inside. Others feel that checking the placenta carefully is all that's needed. If your caregiver does do a manual examination, it can be quite painful, but momentary, and you will have to use your breathing exercises.

Once the placenta is delivered and examined, your caregiver will check your cervix and perineal area for lacerations and will suture them if necessary. If he has performed an episiotomy, this also will be repaired. Local anesthesia, injected into the perineum, is needed for episiotomy repair. During the repair, barring complications, you should be able to hold your baby and to share her with your husband. When the repair is completed, the nurses may tidy you up, wash your perineal area, and perhaps change your gown. Some women experience uncontrollable shaking immediately after delivery or at this time. The shaking is a result of the tremendous physiological changes taking place inside you and is also a result of your supreme effort during first and second stage labor. The shaking usually disappears in a few minutes. If it happens to you, ask for a warm blanket.

If you deliver in a hospital delivery room, you will now be taken to a recovery room, where you will be observed for an hour or two. Many hospitals allow the husband and baby to remain with the mother in the recovery room, and this is something you should find out about well ahead of time. The immediate postpartum period is so special that you should make every effort to stay together. If for some reason you don't make your feelings known beforehand, it's not too late at delivery time. Many parents are so swept away by the labor and birth that they don't think to question the nurses and doctors who bustle around afterward. But if someone is taking your baby away in an isolette or is telling your husband he can't join you in recovery, you can certainly protest. Sometimes hospital personnel are so preoccupied with their own tasks that they don't recognize how important these details are to you. Or they can misinterpret your condition and automatically assume that you're too tired to spend time bonding with your baby, when actually you couldn't settle down unless you did.

If you labor and deliver in a hospital birthing room, you will probably remain there during the recovery period, and you and your husband will have the opportunity to get to know your new baby in a relaxed and comfortable way. If you give birth at an alternative birth center, the three of you will remain together until you leave the center, which is usually about 12 hours after birth.

During the recovery period, the nurses will periodically check your sanitary napkin for signs of excessive bleeding. They will also periodically check your pulse, blood pressure, and temperature and will knead your uterus to encourage it contract down. The kneading can be uncomfortable, and you may perceive it as an assault on your tired body rather than as a necessary procedure. Again, use your breathing techniques.

When the recovery period is over, you will be brought to your room. Depending on the time of day and the hospital's policy, your baby will either be taken to the nursery to be observed or be allowed to remain with you. If the baby is taken to the nursery, your husband may have the option of accompanying her and watching her being weighed and measured and tidied up. Some hospitals will allow both parents and the baby to remain together even after the recovery period if they have taken a private room or if the other bed is unoccupied. "This was a time in our lives when we didn't have money to spend on anything, but as far as we were concerned, there wasn't any better way to spend what we had than to get a private room for the three of us so we could stay together," says one new mother. "We were able to do all those bonding things you read about. We could have, hold, and nurse the baby on demand. It was an incredible experience. We felt so close and wonderful. We went to sleep the first night with my husband holding the baby's hand." This mother, and others who were able to spend time with their husbands and babies after birth, felt that being together was such a powerful force that it carried them through rockier times in the postpartum period when they began their adjustment to new parenthood.

Cesarean Birth

Most women anticipate having a vaginal birth with their husbands present and remaining together afterward with the baby. But for a substantial number of women giving birth each year, a cesarean delivery will be necessary, and this change, especially if it's unexpected, will to some degree affect the nature of the birth experience. Today, however, a cesarean birth, unless it's a rare emergency, can be a family-centered experience as well.

Cesarean rates increased dramatically in the past decade—from approximately 5 percent of all births in 1970 to 16.5 percent in 1980. The current national rate is about 17 to 18 percent, but in some areas and some hospitals it may be even higher. There has been much debate within the medical community about the reasons for this increase. A task force convened by the National Institute of Health (NIH) to study the issue published its conclusions in the fall of 1981.

According to the NIH task force, the single most important cause of the rise in cesarean rates is the general category of dystocia, meaning a difficult or prolonged labor. Cesareans attributed to dystocia account for about 30 percent of the increase. One reason for doing a cesarean in such cases is cephalopelvic disproportion, which is also known as fetopelvic disproportion. Another way of saying this is that the mother's pelvis and the baby do not make a good fit; usually the baby's head is too large to pass through safely. In some labors, uterine contractions may not occur with sufficient frequency or intensity to move the baby along, and this is often referred to as failure to progress. Each physician, however, has his own definition of failure to progress. One may feel that his patients aren't progressing if they haven't dilated within a certain number of hours, while another may give his patients much longer. If a mother isn't progressing, oxytocin may be used to augment labor.

Repeat cesareans account for an additional 25 to 30 percent of the increase. Although traditional obstetric practice is changing in this regard, most women who have had a cesarean delivery will have another with their next child. This reflects the concern of physicians that the scar tissue in the uterus may rupture in active labor. However, the risk of rupture is greatest if a classical cesarean has been performed—a vertical incision in the body of the uterus—and this type of operation is seldom done today. Most cesareans now are low transverse operations—an incision across the lower part of the uterus. The resulting scar is much less likely to rupture.

In view of the major role played by these two categories, the NIH task force recommended that physicians consider them more carefully with the aim of allowing a greater percentage of women to achieve vaginal delivery. As long as no fetal distress is observed in a difficult labor, measures short of surgery can be tried first, such as providing greater emotional support and encouragement, allowing the woman to walk around, to increase her intake of fluids, to rest, or to sleep. To avoid repeat cesareans, a trial of labor can be allowed for selected women who have had a previous low transverse operation, who have no other indications for surgery, and who have rapid access to the appropriate emergency services if required.

Breech presentation and fetal distress each account for another 10 to 15 percent of the increase in the cesarean rate. Nearly all babies are born head first, but other presentations, which are more difficult to manage, occur in 3 or 4 of every 100 births. Breech is the most common, and this means that the baby is lying head up, rather than head down, within the uterus. There are several types of breech presentation: frank, in which the baby sits with his legs straight up; complete, in which the baby sits with legs crossed; and incomplete, in which one or both feet or knees present first. Because of the risks involved—including injury to the baby, as well as prolapse of the umbilical cord, which can cut off the baby's oxygen supply—cesarean section is becoming almost routine for delivery of a breech baby. Physicians who have been trained in vaginal breech deliveries may still perform them if certain criteria are met. Typically, the baby must be in the frank position and his head must not be overextended, his estimated weight must be within the normal range, and the size of the mother's pelvis must be adequate for a vaginal delivery. Fetal distress is usually defined by a continuing drop in the baby's heart beat, indicating that the supply of oxygen is inadequate. It may be associated with a number of different obstetric complications, including dystocia and breech presentation, but it also may happen for reasons that are unclear at the time. A change in the mother's position can sometimes alleviate mild distress, and sometimes the mother is given oxygen to breathe to assist the baby. If fetal distress cannot be reversed, it's a signal for rapid delivery.

The remainder of the rise in the cesarean rate is comprised of a miscellaneous category, ranging from preexisting maternal illness to conditions related directly to the current pregnancy or labor. Maternal diabetes, kidney disease, or an active venereal herpes infection can necessitate a cesarean birth, and the operation may be performed because of premature rupture of the membranes, a postmature pregnancy, or a multiple pregnancy. Not all such problems will inevitably lead to a cesarean, however. In a number of these situations, labor may be induced. Induction is usually accomplished by starting an intravenous drip that contains Pitocin®, a synthetic form of oxytocin, which is the hormone that stimulates labor contractions. Induced contractions begin with a bang, and they're generally stronger, closer together, and peak earlier. This means that they can be more difficult to handle

Childbirth

and require more concentration from a mother and her coach. While induction of labor is an important obstetrical tool, it should never be used solely for convenience. In the past, induction was used quite routinely—babies were born by appointment rather than when they were ready. But induction is not without its risks, which is why it should be used only when medically necessary.

If you learn either during your pregnancy or your labor that a cesarean will be necessary, you will probably feel disappointed. That's only natural. Nevertheless, there are a number of steps you can take to try to ensure that the birth retains some family-centered aspects.

If you know in advance that you will need a cesarean, you will have ample opportunity to discuss the arrangements with your physician. Even if there's no present indication, it's still wise to consider the possibility and to plan the type of delivery you want if complications arise.

Today, many doctors and hospitals recognize the importance of the father's presence during a cesarean delivery—both to share the experience with his wife and to provide invaluable support at a time of emotional stress. Most hospitals will allow the father to be present only if his wife is having regional anesthesia and is awake for the delivery, but some will allow him to witness the birth if she must have general anesthesia. Knowing that your husband saw the delivery and was given the baby to hold can be extremely important to you. If your husband is not permitted in the operating room, the baby can be brought out to him after delivery.

If you are awake and have made the request ahead of time, you may be allowed to nurse the baby right away and to take him with you to recovery where you, your husband, and the baby can spend time getting to know each other. Many hospitals don't allow anyone in surgical recovery except the patient. In that case, try to arrange to be taken to maternity recovery so that your new family doesn't have to be separated.

Even when it is known ahead of time that a cesarean is necessary, a doctor may still wait for labor to begin spontaneously at term, since this is the best way to make sure that the baby is mature enough to be born. If the cesarean must be scheduled more precisely to have the operating room available, it will be on or close to the mother's due date. The baby's status can be assessed by means of ultrasound, which can help determine the baby's age, or by amniocentesis to determine lung maturity.

A cesarean can be performed under regional or general anesthesia. General anesthesia is usually reserved for an emergency. With regional anesthesia, either an epidural or a spinal will be given. The advantage of regional anesthesia, as discussed in the section on childbirth medications, is that you can be awake during the baby's birth and, in most cases, hold or nurse her soon after delivery. With general anesthesia, you will lose consciousness within a few seconds and probably will not awaken until an hour or so after the birth.

The baby is usually born within the first five or ten minutes of the operation. The rest of the time, which is about an hour, is spent in suturing the incisions. Two incisions are made during a cesarean delivery: one in the abdominal wall and another in the uterus. The abdominal incision may not be the same as the uterine incision. They can either be vertical (also called classical or median) or horizontal (also called low transverse or a bikini cut). The

Childbirth

type of abdominal incision should be obvious to you, but the uterine incision will not be and can play a major role in determining what type of birth you will have next time. Ask your doctor if you have any question about it.

Your baby may not be able to stay with you as long as you like after delivery. Some hospitals have a mandatory observation period for cesarean babies—either in the regular nursery or in the intensive care nursery. If your baby is perfectly healthy, this observation period and separation can be frustrating for you. You should make every attempt to visit the baby in the nursery as soon as you feel up to it. If you're planning to breastfeed, make sure your doctor and the nurses know. Pain medication given to you is passed on to the baby through your milk, and your doctor should choose a medication that is least likely to affect the baby.

The traditional hospital stay for a cesarean birth is seven to ten days, but today many women go home earlier if they are comfortable. When you think about going home, remember that you're not just recovering from the birth of a baby, which is quite a task in itself. You're also recovering from surgery and will need extra time to rest and regain your strength.

7. The Postpartum Period

It doesn't always sink in right away, but with the birth of your baby, you have crossed a threshold—you're a parent! As soon as you are handed your baby, the adjustment to parenthood begins. Your body will go through rapid changes starting immediately after birth and continuing for many weeks. And just as it was difficult during pregnancy to separate your emotions from the physical changes taking place, it will be difficult to do so now. Postpartum is every bit the roller coaster that pregnancy was. But the highs are probably even higher and the lows—well, they're equally difficult. One thing is certain, though—the ride you begin once your baby is born lasts more than nine months. It's a marvelous, frightening, delicious, revealing, exasperating, lovely ride for a lifetime.

Your Postpartum Body

The transformation to your pre-pregnant state is faster than your previous metamorphosis into a pregnant woman,

The Postpartum Period

and you may be more uncomfortable in the immediate postpartum period than you expected. "No one talked to me about how much the episiotomy was going to hurt afterwards or how weak I was going to feel," says one new mother. "It didn't last long, but the shock of how I felt was very difficult to handle." Another mother had a similar experience: "I delivered late at night, and when I woke the next morning, I just couldn't believe how awful I felt. It wasn't just the stitches from the episiotomy. My whole body ached. I must have been very tense during the pushing stage and clenched my jaw a lot. It hurt so much the next morning that I really couldn't open it to eat." A third mother remembers getting out of bed the morning after delivery and almost fainting: "No one told me not to get out of bed the first time without a nurse, although I've read this in books since. I was heading toward the bathroom and suddenly everything was swirling. It was over in a minute or two, but I was just amazed." Of course, not all new mothers feel achy, weak, and tired. Some feel terrific. "I expected to want to lie in bed and not move anything," says another new mother. "But I was so excited about seeing the baby again that I jumped up and flew down the hall to the nursery. The stitches never really bothered me, and I simply felt great." How your body feels after birth depends a great deal on the type of labor and delivery you had. It's simply important to know that the immediate postpartum experience can include discomforts so they don't take you by surprise.

Post-Delivery Discomforts

If you had an episiotomy, it may hurt a lot or a little, but there are several things that can be done to help ease the soreness. When you are brought back to your room after the recovery period, you may be given an ice pack for your perineum. This usually makes the area feel much better and reduces swelling, which can make the stitches hurt more. If you aren't given an ice pack, request one from the nurse. Warm sitz baths and heat lamp treatments are also effective in promoting healing and in making you more comfortable. Again, if they aren't offered, be sure to ask for them if you think they'd be helpful. Some caregivers also prescribe medicated sprays or ointments for the episiotomy. You may find it painful to sit for a day or more after delivery. The temptation is to avoid sitting or to sit on something soft. But sitting on a hard chair is actually better for you than sitting on a soft cushion. The cushion may spread the stitches and cause painful pulling. Remember to do your Kegels as soon as possible after delivery. While they're helping to restore tone to your pelvic floor muscles, they can make your episiotomy feel better by restoring blood flow to the area.

You will probably be asked to urinate within a few hours after birth. Urinating may feel strange for a day or two, and you may also feel a burning sensation. The burning doesn't necessarily mean that you have an infection, although urinary tract infections are common after birth. During delivery, the baby pressed rather hard on your bladder and urethra, irritating both. Urine, particularly concentrated urine, will irritate them further and cause the burning sensation. Drinking a lot of water or other liquids will help dilute the urine and ease the burning. If it does not subside, let your caregiver know, as you may have an infection. During the first week after the birth, you will also find yourself urinating more frequently, even if you haven't increased your fluid intake. Your body is ridding itself of the extra water that accumulated in body tissues during pregnancy.

Nurses and doctors in the hospital will probably make a big fuss about your having a bowel movement. You'll be asked often whether or not you've had one, and a stool softener or laxative may be prescribed. While their concern can be irritating, their feeling is that it's better for you to have a bowel movement while you're in the hospital than to wait until you get home. They reason that you'll be afraid of having the first movement because you're so tender in that area (they're right!) and may end up becoming constipated, which will make it even more difficult for you to have a movement.

Throughout pregnancy, your body is producing increased amounts of certain hormones. After delivery, production drops dramatically, and it will take a while for hormonal levels to stabilize. Until they do, you may find yourself sweating more than usual, having periods of hot flashes or flushes, and awakening damp or wringing wet during the night. To cope with night sweats, have enough fresh nightclothes and nursing bras, if you're nursing, so that you can change into something dry and clean.

The Shape of Things to Come

Right after delivery, you will probably look as if you are four or five months pregnant. But don't despair! The uterus begins to shrink as soon as the placenta is delivered and will become progressively smaller and lower. By the end of the first week, the uterus may have descended so far into the pelvic cavity that you may no longer be able to feel it externally. By the end of the fifth or sixth week, it will have completely returned to its pre-pregnant size and weight. This process is known as involution, and the contractions that are part of it can be quite intense at the beginning, especially if this is not your first baby. If you are breastfeeding, you will also be more aware of these so-called afterpains. When the baby suckles, the hormone oxytocin is released into your bloodstream, and this hormone causes the uterus to contract. Nursing, in fact, can help hasten the involution process. If you find the contractions painful, try doing your childbirth breathing exercises.

Your abdomen will be rather lax and flabby, but it will gradually regain muscle tone and elasticity. A regular exercise program can help you get back to pre-pregnancy form, but a strenuous regimen should not be started immediately. The main thing during the postpartum period is to rest and recuperate.

If you take into account the combined weight of the baby, placenta, and amniotic fluid, you can expect to lose between 11 and 13 pounds right after delivery. Over the next few weeks, you will lose additional weight as the body sheds excess fluids and the uterus shrinks. By the end of the postpartum period, you may find that you're only 5 to 10 pounds above your pre-pregnancy weight. With attention to exercise and sound nutrition, most women are back to pre-pregnancy form by three to six months after birth. Proper nutrition is very important during the postpartum period. Just as during pregnancy, you should eat a well-balanced diet drawn from the four basic food groups.

Lochia

This is the term used for the postpartum bleeding and discharge that begins right after delivery. During the first couple of days, the bleeding can be quite heavy, but it will gradually decrease as the walls of the uterus heal. The color of lochia usually changes from bright red to pink or brown, and it may become yellow or white before it disappears completely, which is usually within three or four weeks. If the lochia suddenly becomes heavy and red again after diminishing, it may mean that the former site of the placenta has reopened, probably because you are being too active and not getting enough rest. You should let your physician or nurse-midwife know if this happens.

The Postpartum Checkup

This is usually scheduled four to six weeks after delivery. Your caregiver will do a pelvic examination to be sure that the uterus has returned to its pre-pregnancy size and location, and she will check the condition of your episiotomy, if you had one. Your breasts and abdomen will be examined, your weight will be recorded, and your blood pressure will be measured.

New mothers are usually advised not to have sexual intercourse until after the postpartum checkup. This is to ensure that the episiotomy has healed properly and the cervix has closed. You should discuss family planning methods with your caregiver during this checkup. If you are breastfeeding, you may not begin to menstruate until you have weaned your baby. But while breastfeeding delays the onset of menstruation, it is not a guarantee against conception. You may begin ovulating before you get your first period. Many babies have been conceived as a result of "nature's contraceptive," as some people call the absence of periods while nursing. If you are bottle-feeding, you may begin to menstruate six to eight weeks after birth.

The postpartum checkup is also a good time to ask your caregiver about starting a regular exercise program, if you haven't asked already. It can be hard to follow an exercise regimen with a new baby in the house, so once you've gotten your caregiver's okay, you may want to join a postpartum exercise class. Some of the organizations that offer postpartum classes also provide free baby-sitting or baby-sitting for a nominal fee. Getting out and doing something for yourself will probably do you a lot of good.

Your Postpartum Self

How you feel emotionally during the first days and weeks after birth will probably change hourly. Your feelings will be affected by your birth experience, by the support you get or don't get from your husband, family, and friends, by hormonal changes, and, of course, by your baby. Some mothers are surprised by the intensity of their feelings after birth. They feel high, elated, ecstatic. "I remember thinking I had just done the neatest thing I could ever possibly do," says one new mother. Others are surprised by how little they feel. "I was totally numb. After all those hours in labor, I looked at the baby and wondered what he was doing there," says another mother.

Try not to have expectations on your emotions. If you expect to feel euphoric when the baby's born and you don't, it doesn't mean there's something wrong with you. It takes time to get used to being a parent—even though you've been planning it for nine months. So much has happened to you in such a short amount of time—discovering you were in labor and then getting through it—that you are in a state of emotional crisis already when the baby is born.

Fathers, too, can experience either side of the emotional spectrum. Some fathers are overcome with emotion as their children are born, crying tears of joy. Others feel distant from their babies and are primarily relieved that labor and delivery are over. Parents who are able to spend time together and with their newborns after delivery generally have better feelings about each other and their babies. "I never felt anything but terrific emotionally," says one new mother. "But I think it's because my husband was there at the time, in recovery, and in my room until we went home."

You may not immediately fall in love with your baby. Everyone thinks that it will be love at first sight, but it isn't always so. If you had a difficult labor and delivery, you may need time to feel sorry about it, and you may be distracted by pain or your unrealized expectations. You may even resent your baby for causing all the trouble. You may suddenly feel sad about having lost the happy time of your pregnancy. One mother of a three-month-old says, "I still have moments of thinking, gee, I'm not special. I'm not pregnant anymore. But being pregnant is not more neat than having the baby on the outside playing with you in the bathtub."

Keep in mind that the baby is primarily a stranger to you. That's an odd thought, since he's your child and you've been carrying him inside you for nine months. But he's someone you've never set eyes on before. Even if you feel very close to him right away, there is a getting-to-know-you period that can last for some time after the birth. You may be surprised by how the baby looks— you may have thought you'd have a brunette and ended up with a blonde, or you may have been sure you were having a girl and instead you produced a boy. Not only will the baby be physically different from what you expected, you may have feelings about the differences. One new mother remembers being confused at the nursery window the first time she went to take a peek at her son. "I was wide awake and alert for the birth and held my son for about half an hour that night. And yet the next morning when I went to see him, I wasn't quite sure which one was mine," she says. "It was a very eerie feeling."

It's important during the postpartum period that you talk about how you're feeling—especially with your husband, but also with family and friends and with other new mothers you meet in the hospital. Talking will help you clarify your feelings and will make others aware of your needs. In particular, keep the lines of communication open with your husband. Chances are he's having a lot of roller-coaster feelings too and with precious few people to share them with.

Going Home

This is when you stop playing at being a parent and actually become one. It's when the awesome weight of responsibility suddenly hits you. One new mother remembers sitting in the hospital bathroom in labor after having had an enema and thinking, "Oh, God, what did I get myself into?" That same feeling—of fear, of not being able to turn back or to stop and change your mind—may occur or reoccur when you bring the baby home.

In the hospital, there was always someone to ask when you didn't know how to diaper or if you were breast-feeding properly. And you could always tuck the baby into her bassinet and take her back to the nursery when you were feeling a little overwhelmed or tired or when you just wanted to take a breather. At home, unless you hired help or have a friend or relative lending a hand during the first week or so, it's you and your husband who will be assuming full-time care of the baby. You will undoubtedly be scared and unsure of yourselves.

But going home is also the most exciting and electrifying time. It's the culmination of your months of planning and dreaming. It's when you get to use the little baby clothes and blankets that you weren't ever really convinced you'd need. Especially after a hospital stay, you probably will be anxious to get home and settled.

Postpartum Blues

This is a term used to pinpoint feelings of dejection that may occur either fleetingly or for a day, a few days, or even a week or more. Not everyone experiences postpartum blues. Of the women who responded to the *Parents* childbirth poll, 55 percent said they did. Why some women do and others don't is unclear and probably depends on many factors. Hormonal changes are often blamed, at least in part, for the postpartum blues. But there's little doubt that the upheaval that your baby's birth causes in your life is primarily responsible. If you don't become depressed, terrific! If you do, try to relax and remember that this too will pass. And you have every right to your feelings. A baby is a big responsibility, something that's difficult to appreciate until you actually have one. Suddenly you can't leave the house spontaneously or without your constant companion. If you haven't been around children or babies before, the simplest baby care duties may seem like grave tasks. Putting on a diaper may be a challenge, as may burping and bathing and dressing. And you may be concerned that you're not doing these things the right way. (Keep telling yourself that there is

The Postpartum Period

no right way, as long as the baby gets fed, dressed, and changed.) You'll wonder if you'll ever feel competent at this baby business. If your life was well organized before, it suddenly won't be for a while. Dinner may not get cooked or it will get burned, the baby may cry her way through your mealtimes so that you and your husband never get a chance to sit down together, and cooking and cleaning may seem like impossibilities on top of the other things you're doing.

The type of baby you have will also affect how you feel. Some parents luck out with babies who sleep a lot and cry a little. Others have babies who don't sleep much or who sleep at odd and inconvenient hours or who cry incessantly. If you don't get much sleep at night, you'll be tired during the day, and exhaustion can play a role in depression too. When you're tired, it's harder to handle anything, especially this new parenting job. Try to sleep when the baby sleeps, if you can, so you'll get enough rest. "Everybody was telling me to lie down as soon as the baby went to sleep," says one new mother. "It seemed like sage but impossible advice. How could I sleep when I was anxious about everything: about when the baby was going to wake me, about when I was going to make dinner, go grocery shopping, write thank-you notes. It took me weeks to calm down and do what they suggested. But you know, once I did it, it was great. I had to plan my other times better, get more organized—or do the opposite and just let everything go. But the sleep I got was the most important ingredient in my mental and physical health."

Taking the phone off the hook or unplugging it is a trick for peace and quiet that many new mothers learn once they're home. You can also leave a note on your doorbell to keep people from ringing or visiting when the baby is sleeping and you're napping, or if you're feeding the baby and don't want to be disturbed. Visitors can be a blessing at times, or they can be a real nuisance. It's very difficult to know yourself how much is too much visiting. You'll be eager to show off your baby and to see friends and family, and it's easy to overdo it and exhaust yourself. You may find it hard or next to impossible to say no to a request for a visit, even if you know that it's too much for you. Especially in the beginning, have your husband field visiting requests. It may be easier for him to say to your cousin, "You know, we'd love to see you, but Susie is completely exhausted right now. Why don't you try us next week?" He'll probably win the husband of the year award, and you'll get the rest you need.

You and your husband will be insecure about the job you're doing as new parents, and you may be very sensitive to suggestions from each other. After exhausting days of baby care and nights of interrupted sleep, you may find that you are communicating less, even arguing. Having a new baby is stressful. The most important thing you can do during this time is to summon up the extra bit of energy it takes to talk with your husband about how you're feeling and to ask him about how he's feeling, if he doesn't volunteer the information. This means sharing the euphoria as well as the insecurity, the fun as well as the fear. You need to care about each other physically as well as emotionally, to show that you love each other by touching too, although that may be difficult at first.

Sex

Asked about sex in the postpartum period, one mother of a three-month-old laughed and said, "I'm sure the section you write on that is going to be very short!" Her experience of infrequent sex and a diminished sex drive is very common among new mothers and fathers. There are physical and emotional reasons for a decreased desire for sex, if you experience it. Physically, you are recuperating from birth. Your caregiver will probably advise that you not have sexual intercourse for four to six weeks, or until after you have been examined at the postpartum checkup. Fatigue also plays a big part in diminished interest in sex. New parents are tired parents, both because of the 'round-the-clock attention a newborn needs and because of the effort required to adjust emotionally to parenthood.

You and your husband may also be very worried about the baby interrupting your tryst, even if you do get in the mood and find a quiet time and place. It's hard to feel sexy when you're listening with one ear for the baby to cry. Babies seem to have an uncanny way of screaming for attention just when their parents are finally getting a chance to love each other. Try planning a special time to make love—even if planning itself seems unromantic. Perhaps your baby usually naps at a certain time. Try feeding him and putting him down for a nap. Knowing that his tummy is satisfied may make you feel more at ease.

Your first sessions of lovemaking will take time and

patience on both your parts. You'll probably be very nervous about how intercourse will feel. You may fear pain; your husband may fear hurting you. The vagina will probably be drier than it was before birth, and penetration may be difficult. Vaginal dryness is apparently due to the hormonal imbalance that follows childbirth. The problem is temporary, although it usually lasts longer among nursing mothers. Spend a lot of time in foreplay so that your vagina will become lubricated or have your husband apply a lubricant before penetration. When he enters you, he should do so very slowly and gently. If you feel pain or you're not ready, that's okay. You may need to do this several times before you actually make love. Pain with the first intercourse or two is common, but if it persists, you should consult your physician or nurse-midwife.

Oftentimes, women spend so much of their day loving and nurturing their babies that they feel they have little left for their husbands. This may be hard for your husband to understand. He needs love and affection from you as well, and the two of you need to show each other love by touching as well as through words. You also need to be loved physically by your husband so that you will be able to love your baby. You can't always just give; you must also receive. "The first couple of months, it was a shock to hug each other, because we were so big," recalls one mother. "But those big-people hugs can go a long way!"

Not everyone needs to work at sexual loving after they have a child. Some couples find that their sexual relationship is better than ever and does not decline after the baby is born. For the majority, though, having a baby temporarily disturbs their sexual relationship. But with time and good communication, the difficulties are overcome and sex is once again integrated into your relationship as a whole.

Adjusting to being a parent is probably the most challenging and ongoing task you will be confronted with. It will bring you more pleasure and joy, more confidence (even in your uncertainty), more zest for life, and sensitivity to yourself and others. It's hard to have perspective when you are going through the initial adjustment period. If you feel overwhelmed now, you can be sure it won't last. You won't recognize yourself or your baby in a couple of months. "I was so afraid that having a baby would spoil everything or change things too much," says one mother of a four-month-old. "But I'm finding that it enhances everything—me, my marriage. What else could you do that's better?"

Your Newborn

Your baby may look like you or your husband or like no relative you ever saw. He may bear more resemblance to a prize fighter after the championship bout than to any member of your family tree. But to you he will be the most adorable and brilliant child ever born. It's every parent's inalienable right to believe in the perfection of her creation.

Appearance

If you've never seen a newborn, you may be surprised by your baby's appearance at birth. His head will be quite large compared to the rest of his body, and it may be "molded" or elongated. The baby's skull bones do not fuse before birth so that they can overlap and allow the head to pass safely through the birth canal. As a result, the head is usually elongated and somewhat pointed in back. Unless your baby is born with a thick head of hair, you will probably notice a soft spot on the top of his head. This is the largest of the fontanels, the places where the skull bones are not yet fused, and it is covered with a thick protective membrane.

Some newborns have lots of hair, some have little, and some have none. "I remember how excited the nurses were when my son was born," recalls one mother. "He had long, thick hair that they could comb and even part. He still wears his hair parted the same way they did it in the hospital!" Regardless of how much hair your baby has or doesn't have at birth, his hair may be quite different several months hence. The hair a baby is born with is gradually shed and replaced by the permanent hair, which can be an entirely different color and texture. The color of your baby's eyes may also change. Most babies have gray-blue eyes at birth, and the permanent color usually doesn't become evident until about six months.

Your baby will probably enter the world covered with vernix caseosa, a whitish, creamy substance that protects the skin before birth. You may also notice a fine fuzz on his shoulders, back, ears, cheeks, and forehead. This hair is called lanugo and will gradually disappear. Babies born prematurely often have more lanugo than babies born near or at term. Lanugo has no relation to how much hair your baby will have later in life or to whether he will have thick body hair as an adult. Your new baby will probably be looking red for a while, and his skin will be fairly trans-

The Postpartum Period

parent. His complexion may be mottled, and there may be a number of spots and blemishes, which will gradually disappear. In a month or two, his complexion will begin to look more like what you probably envisioned—velvety smooth and blemish-free.

A baby's genitals are often swollen at birth—a boy's scrotum and a girl's vulva will look disproportionately large. Both boys and girls may have swollen breasts, and the nipples may even secrete tiny amounts of milk. Girls often have a whitish vaginal discharge, which may be tinged with blood. All of these are the result of maternal hormones that entered the baby's bloodstream before birth, and they will gradually subside and disappear.

Senses

Your baby is born with well-developed senses. She can see, hear, taste, smell, and feel you touch her from birth. Of all the senses, sight is the least mature. Your baby will see at birth but not as well as you. Her eyes focus best at about 8 to 12 inches. She can distinguish color and pattern, can follow a slowly moving object, and will prefer to look at a pattern that resembles the human face. Newborns are also sensitive to light and will squint or close their eyes in bright light.

When she is born, your baby will have been hearing sounds for quite some time—both the sounds within your body and some sounds from outside the womb. She will alert to the sound of the human voice and prefer it to other sounds. She will prefer high-pitched voices to low ones. When she hears a new sound, a baby will momentarily stop nursing to listen. Newborns also like rhythm—the ticking of a clock, for instance.

Just like you, your baby prefers sweet tastes to sour ones. A baby will contort her face after tasting something bitter but will suck longest, when given a choice, on a bottle containing sweet liquid. Babies also dislike strong odors and will cry. A baby's sense of smell is so acute that she can differentiate the smell of her own mother's milk from another mother's.

The baby's sense of touch is his most highly developed sense. Babies love to be held, touched gently, swaddled. This loving handling communicates your feelings to him and gives him a sense of well-being. This touching is so important that babies who have been institutionalized and deprived of touching often have developmental delays and are more sickly than their peers from loving homes.

Reflexes

Your baby will also come equipped with a variety of reflexes. The feeding reflexes are among those necessary to her survival. The most immediately obvious of these is the rooting reflex. If you touch or stroke her cheek, the baby will turn her head automatically in that direction and move her mouth, looking for the nipple to latch on to. When the baby does suck, she will swallow, but the gag reflex will prevent her from choking if she takes too big a gulp. Breathing is another reflex that's essential for survival. Sneezing, coughing, and yawning serve useful purposes as well. Sneezing and coughing clear the airways of mucus, and yawning increases the baby's oxygen supply when she needs it.

Crying is a reflex and a primitive form of communication. Whenever your baby cries, she is trying to tell you that something is bothering her. She may be hungry or wet or simply bored. Whatever the reason, you should respond promptly to her cries. Babies who are responded to quickly feel loved and often cry less as they mature than babies who are left to cry it out. After a while, you'll be able to distinguish between a hunger cry, a cry of pain, or a cry of irritability. Babies' chins and lower lips often tremble when they cry. Although it can look frightening, it's normal.

Some of your baby's reflexes are holdovers from earlier days and serve no useful purpose now. The grasp reflex, in which the baby firmly grasps an object that strokes her palm, is one example. Another example is the Moro reflex (also called the startle reflex). The baby will react to any loud noise or sudden, jerky movement by flinging his arms out wide and then bringing them together in an embrace position. The baby may also cry when startled.

Several other reflexes are the forerunners of skills he will learn later. Some examples of these are the stepping reflex and the crawling reflex. If you hold the baby upright and touch his feet to a flat, firm surface, he will move his legs and feet, as if he were stepping. Many new parents delight in this stepping and don't realize that it's a reflex that will fade. It does not indicate that the baby will be an early walker. Similarly, if you place the baby on his stomach, he may lift his head and make crawling movements.

The tonic neck reflex, also called the fencing reflex, helps the baby learn about spatial relationships and may be an early indicator of hand preference. In this reflex, the baby turns his head to one side. The arm on that side is outstretched. The arm on the opposite side is flexed and the fist is near the back of the head.

Sleeping and Feeding

During the hospital stay, your baby will probably sleep a lot and cry a little, but this pattern may change dramatically once you get home. New parents often find this sudden change disconcerting. In the hospital, the baby seemed so "good," and now she cries a lot and sleeps in spurts. The change can make you feel incompetent or like you're doing something to make the baby unhappy. The simple truth is, however, that during the first few days, a baby normally sleeps a lot, as she recoups from the stress of birth and the initial adjustment from uterine to outside life. By the time you go home, she is starting to emerge from this period of "R and R" and is establishing a more normal life for herself—although what's normal for her may seem abnormal to you!

A newborn usually sleeps about 14 to 18 hours a day. That seems like a lot, and it is. But she may not spend those hours sleeping at night or sleeping for hours at a time. If you have a baby who dozes for 20 minutes, then wakes and cries, then dozes again, it can be very frustrating. "It seemed that as soon as I got started doing something after he fell asleep, he was up again," says one new mother. "I never got to finish the dishes, I left hand

The Postpartum Period

laundry half-rinsed in the sink, and I was scared to death to take a shower, because he might wake up when I had just started soaping." If you have a baby like this, a soft front carrier can be a blessing. The baby may sleep longer or be more content if she is snuggled against you, and you'll be able to get some chores done.

Irregularity is to be expected with feeding times too. While some babies have little trouble adapting to a regular schedule, most need time before they settle into a fairly predictable feeding routine. You will be feeding your baby often during the newborn period. Especially if you are breastfeeding, you may find that your baby wants to nurse every two hours during the early weeks. Breast milk is very easy to digest, and a new baby needs small, frequent feedings throughout the day. And you will need these frequent nursings to help establish your milk supply. Formula takes longer to digest, and a bottle-fed baby may be able to go longer between feedings—perhaps three or four hours. Flexibility is the guide word when it comes to new-baby care. Says one new mother, "I've never been a very flexible person, but the baby has literally forced me to become one. Now that I can be easier about when he eats and sleeps, I find I'm more flexible in other areas of my life as well." As your baby's systems mature, she will become more regular in her routines. The number of hours she sleeps each day will gradually decrease, and she will begin sleeping for longer periods of time. The number of feedings will also decrease, and there will be more time between those feedings.

Bathing

Newborn babies don't get dirty all over so there's no reason to give them a full-fledged sponge bath or tub bath every day. You should, however, be sure to keep the face and neck creases clean, and to thoroughly cleanse the diaper area after each bowel movement.

Your pediatrician will probably advise you to give your baby a sponge bath until the umbilical stump has fallen off. You will be told to keep the umbilical area clean (usually you'll dab it with some alcohol after every diaper change) and dry, keeping the diaper fastened below it. When the stump falls off, you may see a few spots of blood or a tiny discharge. This is normal. If you see further discharge or bleeding, call your doctor. Your baby could have an infection.

Once the stump has fallen off, you can give your baby a real bath. If you're scared, wait until your husband is home so you can do it together, or ask a friend or relative to come help. Gather all the bath items *before* you undress the baby or put him in the tub. Never leave a baby unattended in the bath even for a second.

When giving a bath, talk or sing to the baby to make him comfortable. Newborns often hate getting undressed and scream unless they are wrapped and secure in your arms. They still are more used to the feeling of snugness they had in the womb than to the feeling of being totally exposed. Your baby may not like the bath for a while. If he doesn't, there's no reason to keep him in there long or to bathe him every day. As he gets older, he'll like it more and more. "My son hated the bath until he was about three months old, but I felt I had to give him one every day," says one mother. "I was really embarrassed when a neighbor asked what I did to him every day at seven P.M. that made him scream. I'm not sure she believed me when I told her it was his bath time!" And one pediatrician says you can tell how many children a mother has by how often she bathes the baby. New mothers bathe their babies every day, he says. Mothers with more than one child don't.

In these first weeks, you will have a lot to learn about baby care and about your individual baby. There will be many firsts, many surprises. With each feeding, bath, each playtime with your baby, you will discover more things about her, get to know her better, and become more comfortable in caring for her. As you are learning about your role as a parent, your baby will be growing and changing too. Soon you will be settled into a routine of ever-changing routines. Soon you will look back on this newborn period with a smile.

Afterword

When you have a baby, you haven't just added a person to your household. You have changed your household's very nature. You were a couple. Now you are a family.

You may not have given much thought to the idea of family before—even though when you and your husband decided to have a baby, you may have told each other, or been told by others, that "now is the time to start a family." The dynamics of family life are different from those of a couple. Although you've only added one person to the household, the number of relationships in it have multiplied exponentially. There's your marital relationship, your relationship to your child, your husband's relationship to his child, and your relationship to each other as parents.

Your relationship to the rest of the world changes as well. You are now seen not solely in terms of yourself as an individual or as part of a married couple, but as a parent. You may be treated as more responsible, with more respect, than you ever were before. And you certainly will receive society's approval for reproducing and

Afterword

settling down to the business of raising the next generation.

Your relationship with your parents will continue to change, as it began to during pregnancy. It's an odd feeling to be both child and parent. Your parents may also feel strange relating to you as a parent and as a child. In a sense, you are on equal footing. As you begin to take care of your new baby, you may suddenly realize all the ways your parents must have nurtured you, and you may have a strong feeling of identification with them for the first time. It may be a revelation to you that your parents, like you, struggled through learning to change a diaper, through fevers, rashes, sleepless nights, and insecurities, that at one time they didn't know any more than you do about baby care. You may forgive them their shortcomings in a much bigger way than you did during pregnancy.

The feeling of being a family doesn't happen all at once. It's a gradual evolution. Your inner picture of family life (kids, pets, laughter all jumbled up) may seem a far cry from the tableau at your house right now (bed unmade, baby spit-up dribbling down your blouse, exhausted father falling asleep in front of the TV). But all these pictures are what family is made of. Family is eating out for the first time after the birth with the baby fast asleep in his infant seat; it's strolling together so proudly down the street with the baby in his carriage, changing diapers in strange restaurant and park bathrooms, sharing the midnight feeding shift, eating meals with baby in one hand and fork in the other. It's sharing all the firsts, the laughter and tears, the feeling deep in the pit of your stomach that you haven't the vaguest idea what you're doing or what you should be doing. Family is everyone snuggling together in bed for another few minutes' snooze, that indescribably sweet warmth and closeness of baby breath and baby fuzz between you. Your numbers have increased; parents and baby are growing. Welcome to the beginning

Bibliography of Further Reading

Pregnancy and Birth

Birth Without Violence, Frederick Leboyer. Alfred A. Knopf, 1975.

Changing Childbirth: Family Birth in the Hospital, Diony Young. Childbirth Graphics Ltd., 1982.

Childbirth: A Source Book for Conception, Pregnancy, Birth and the First Weeks of Life, Sharron Hannon. M. Evans and Company, 1980.

Chidbirth With Love: A Complete Guide to Fertility, Pregnancy, and Childbirth for Caring Couples, Niels H. Lauersen, M.D. G. P. Putnam's Sons, 1983.

The Complete Book of Pregnancy and Childbirth, Sheila Kitzinger. Alfred A. Knopf, 1983.

The Gentle Birth Book, Nancy Berezin. Simon and Schuster, 1980.

Have It Your Way, Vicki E. Walton. Bantam Books, 1978.

The New Pregnancy, Susan S. Lichtendorf and Phyllis L. Gillis. Bantam Books, 1981.

Rights of the Pregnant Parent, Valmai Howe Elkins. Schocken Books, 1980.

Childbirth Alternatives

The Complete Book of Midwifery, Barbara Brennan, C.N.M., and Joan R. Heilman. E. P. Dutton, 1977.
Immaculate Deception, Suzanne Arms. Bantam Books, 1977.
NAPSAC Directory of Alternative Birth Services and Consumer Guide, Penny Simkin, with revisions and additions by Jamy Braun and Lee Stewart, 1982.

Nutrition

As You Eat, So Your Baby Grows: A Guide to Nutrition in Pregnancy, Nikki Goldbeck. A pamphlet published by Ceres Press, Box 87, Dept. D., Woodstock, New York 12498.
Caring for Your Unborn Child, Ronald E. Gots, M.D., and Barbara A. Gots, M.D. Bantam Books, 1979.
Pickles & Ice Cream: The Complete Guide to Nutrition During Pregnancy, Mary Abbot Hess, R.D., and Anne Elise Hunt. McGraw-Hill, 1982.
What Every Pregnant Woman Should Know: The Truth About Diets and Drugs in Pregnancy, Gail Sforza Brewer with Tom Brewer, M.D. Random House, 1977.

Exercise

The Complete Pregnancy Exercise Program, Diana Simkin. New American Library, 1980.
Essential Exercises for the Childbearing Year, Elizabeth Noble. Houghton Mifflin, 1982.
The Exercise Plus Pregnancy Program, Lazar and Olinda Cedeno and Carol Monroe. William Morrow and Co., 1980.
Jane Fonda's Workout Book for Pregnancy, Birth, and Recovery, Femmy DeLyser. Simon and Schuster, 1982.

Emotions

The Experience of Childbirth, Sheila Kitzinger. Penguin Books, 1981.
Making Love During Pregnancy, Elisabeth Bing and Libby Colman. Bantam Books, 1977.
Pregnancy: The Psychological Experience, Arthur and Libby Colman. Bantam Books, 1977.

Fathers

Becoming a Father: A Handbook for Expectant Fathers, Sean Gresh. Butterick Publishing, 1980.
Expectant Fathers, Sam Bittman and Sue Rosenberg Zalk, Ph.D. Ballantine Books, 1980.

The Father Book: Pregnancy and Beyond, Rae Grad et al. Acropolis Books, 1981.
Pregnant Fathers, Jack Heinowitz. Prentice-Hall, 1982.

Prepared Childbirth

Childbirth Without Fear, Grantly Dick-Read, M.D.; revised and edited by Helen Wessel and Harlan F. Ellis, M.D. Harper & Row, 1984.
Husband-Coached Childbirth, Robert A. Bradley, M.D. Harper & Row, 1981.
Six Practical Lessons for an Easier Childbirth, Elisabeth Bing. Bantam Books, 1977.
Thank You, Dr. Lamaze, Marjorie Karmel. Harper & Row, 1981.

Cesarean Birth

Cesarean Birth: A Couple's Guide for Decision and Preparation, Kathleen Mitchell and Marty Nason, R.N. Harbor Publishing, 1981.
Cesarean Childbirth: A Handbook for Parents, Christine Coleman Wilson and Wendy Roe Hovey. Dolphin Books, 1980.
Impact of Cesarean Childbirth, Dyanne Affonso. F. A. Davis Co., 1980.
Silent Knife: Cesarean Prevention and Vaginal Birth After Cesarean, Nancy Wainer Cohen and Lois J. Estner. Bergin & Garvey Publications, 1983.

Bibliography of Further Reading

Postpartum

The Fourth Trimester: On Becoming a Mother, Brenda Krause Eheart and Susan Karol Martel. Appleton-Century-Crofts, 1983.

Living With Your New Baby: A Postpartum Guide for Mothers and Fathers, Elly Rakowitz and Gloria S. Rubin. Franklin Watts, Inc., 1978.

Now That You've Had Your Baby, Gideon G. Panter, M.D., and Shirley M. Linde. Prentice-Hall, 1977.

Breastfeeding

The Complete Book of Breastfeeding, Marvin S. Eiger, M.D., and Sally Wendkos Olds. Workman Publishing, 1972.

The Experience of Breastfeeding, Sheila Kitzinger. Penguin Books, 1980.

Parents™ Book of Breastfeeding, Susan Flamholtz Trien. Ballantine Books, 1983.

The Womanly Art of Breastfeeding, La Leche League International, 1981.

Infant Care and Development

Baby and Child Care, Benjamin Spock, M.D. Pocket Books, 1976.

The First Twelve Months of Life, edited by Frank Caplan. Bantam Books, 1978.

The Mothers' and Fathers' Medical Encyclopedia, Virginia E. Pomeranz, M.D., and Dodi Schultz. New American Library, 1978.

Parents® Book for Your Baby's First Year, Maja Bernath. Ballantine Books, 1983.

Special Situations

After a Loss in Pregnancy, Nancy Berezin. Simon and Schuster, 1982.

Having Twins: A Parent's Guide to Pregnancy, Birth and Early Parenthood, Elizabeth Noble. Houghton Mifflin, 1980.

The Premie Parents Handbook: A Lifeline for the New Parents of a Premature Baby, Adrienne B. Lieberman and Thomas G. Sheagran, M.D. E. P. Dutton, 1984.

Safe Delivery: Protecting Your Baby During High Risk Pregnancy, Roger Freeman, M.D., and Susan C. Pescar. McGraw-Hill, 1983.

You Can Breastfeed Your Baby...Even in Special Situations, Dorothy Patricia Brewster. Rodale Press, 1979.

The following carry publications of interest to pregnant couples and new parents. Write for their catalogs:

Birth and Life Bookstore, P. O. Box 70625, Seattle, Washington 98107.

Bibliography of Further Reading

International Childbirth Education Association (ICEA), P.O. Box 20048, Minneapolis, Minnesota 55420.

Maternity Center Association, 48 E. 92 St., New York, New York 10028.

the penny press, 1100 23rd Ave., Seattle, Washington 98112.

The Resource Center, American College of Obstetricians and Gynecologists, 600 Maryland Ave., S.W., Washington, D.C. 20024 (include a stamped, self-addressed envelope).

Organizations for Expectant Parents

Childbirth Alternatives

American College of Home Obstetrics, P.O. Box 25, River Forest, Illinois 60305.

American College of Nurse-Midwives, 1522 K St., N.W., Suite 1120, Washington, D.C. 20005.

Home Oriented Maternity Experience (HOME), 511 New York Ave., Takoma Park, Washington, D.C. 20012.

National Association of Childbearing Centers, Box 1, Route 1, Perkiomenville, Pennsylvania 18074.

National Association of Parents and Professionals for Safe Alternatives in Childbirth (NAPSAC), P.O. Box 267, Marble Hill, Missouri 63764.

Prepared Childbirth

American Academy of Husband-Coached Childbirth (AAHCC), P.O. Box 5224, Sherman Oaks, California 91413.

American Society for Psychoprophylaxis in Obstetrics (ASPO), 1840 Wilson Blvd., Suite 204, Arlington, Virginia 22201.

International Childbirth Education Association (ICEA), P.O. Box 20048, Minneapolis, Minnesota 55420.

Cesarean Birth

Cesarean/Support, Education and Concern (C/SEC), 22 Forest Road, Framingham, Massachusetts 01701.

Breastfeeding

La Leche League International, 9616 Minneapolis Ave., Franklin Park, Illinois 60131.

Special Situations

Compassionate Friends, P.O. Box 1347, Oak Brook, Illinois 60521 (for bereaved parents).

March of Dimes Birth Defects Foundation, 1275 Mamaroneck Ave., White Plains, New York 10605.

National Organization of Mothers of Twins Clubs, 5402 Amberwood Lane, Rockville, Maryland 20853.

Parents of Premature and High Risk Infants International, Maureen Lynch, Executive Director, c/o The National Self-Help Clearinghouse, 33 W. 42 St., New York, New York 10036.

Index

Abdominal pain, 99
Abruptio placenta, 103–104
   cigarette smoking and, 88
Active phase of labor, 229–36
Afterpains, 189, 258
Alcohol, use for premature labor, 106
Alcohol use, 89–90
   Fetal Alcohol Syndrome, 89–90
Allergies, breastfeeding and, 188
Alpha-fetoprotein (AFP) Testing, 112
Alternative birth center, 46–50
   Childbearing Center (New York City), 48–49
   early discharge, 19
   low/high risk mothers and, 47–48
   referral source for, 50
   setting, 49–50
   staff of, 47
Amniocentesis, 109–111
   Rh disease and, 111
   when advisable, 110
Amniotic sac
   premature rupturing of, 104–105
   rupturing of, 222–25
Analgesia, 215–16
Anencephaly, test for, 112
Anesthesia, 216–19
   Caesarean birth and, 252
   caudal, 218
   eating/drinking and, 29
   epidural, 217
   general, 216–17
   local, 218
   paracervical block, 218
   perineal block, 218
   pudendal block, 218

regional, 217
spinal, 217–18
Antibodies, 63
Apgar score, 244
Aspirin, 84
Auscultation, 31–32
Auto restraints, choosing, 168–70

Babies, *See* Preparing for baby; Newborns.
Baby seat, choosing, 177–78
Back carriers, choosing, 172
Backache, 69
Bathing
  choosing baby bath, 167–68
  newborns, 276–77
Bicycle riding, 153
Birth defects, drugs and, 81–82
Birth Without Violence (Leboyer), 21
Birthing room, 8–11
  criteria for use of, 9
  reasons for, 8–9
  underutilization of, 9–10
Black, R., 26
Blankets, choosing, 184–85
Bleeding, postpartum (lochia), 259
Blood count, test for, 93–94
Blood type, test for, 93
Bonding, 11–13, 243
  mother/child behavior and, 11–12
  post-delivery routines and, 13
  research on, 11–13
  sensitive period, 11–12
Bottlefeeding, 192–94
  basic equipment, 193
  breast/bottle combination, 194–95
  kinds of formula, 192–93
Bowling, 154
Bradley, R., 206–209
Braxton Hicks contractions, 63, 220
Breastfeeding, 187–92
  advantages of, 188–90
  allergies and, 188
  breast/bottle combination, 194–95
  La Leche League, 190–92
  rooming-in and, 15
Breasts, changes in pregnancy, 59, 61, 63
Breathlessness, 63
Breech presentation, 249–50
Bunting, choosing, 184

Caesarean birth, 247–53
  anesthesia, 252
  breech presentations, 249–50
  cephalopelvic disproportion, 248
  dystocia, 248
  fathers' presence and, 251–52
  incision sites, 249, 252
  reasons for, 248–50
  spinal, 217–18
Caffeine, 85–86

Index

Car seat, choosing, 168–70
Carriage, choosing, 172–74
Caudal, 218
Caul, 225
Cephalopelvic disproportion, 248
Cervix
  active phase of labor and, 229–30
  contractions and, 222
  dilation, 225–26
  first stage of labor, 226
  transition phase, 236
Changing table, choosing, 165–67
Childbearing Center (CbC), 48–49
Childbirth, 202–53
  Caesarean birth, 247–53
  complications, 100–107
  contractions, 222, 225–26, 229–30, 236, 239
  labor, 219–47
  medication, 213–19
  prepared childbirth, 203–213
Childbirth care
  alternative birth center, 46–50
  decision-making about, 4–5, 33–42
  family-centered care, 6–8
  homebirth, 50–53
  nurse-midwife, 42–46
  physician/hospital care, 21–33
  referral sources, 33–36
Childbirth Without Fear
(Dick-Read), 205
Cigarette smoking, 86–89
  childhood disorders and, 88
  low birth weight and, 87
Colostrum, 63, 188
Complications, 100–107
  abruptio placenta, 103–104
  placentia previa, 103–104
  postmature syndrome, 107
  premature labor, 105–107
  premature rupture of the membranes, 104–105
  Rh disease, 100–101
  toxemia, 102–103
Constipation, 57, 67–68
  relief of, 67–68
Consultations, 37–42
  advantages of, 38–39
  questions to ask during, 39–41
  sensitivity toward doctor, 39
Contractions
  active phase of labor, 229
  Braxton Hicks contractions, 63
  delivery of placenta, 244
  early, 225
  first stage of labor, 226, 229–30
  purpose of, 222
  second stage of labor, 239
  in transition phase, 236
Couvade syndrome, 118
Crib
  bumpers, 185
  choosing, 162–65
  crib sheets, 185

mattress pad, 185
Crying, newborn, 273

Demerol, 215
Depression, postpartum, 264–66
Diabetes, gestational, 93
Diapers, choosing, 182–83
Dick-Read, G., 204–205
Diet, 75–80
  fruits/vegetables, 77
  grains, 77
  liquids, 77–78
  milk/dairy products, 76–77
  nutritional supplements, 78–80
  protein foods, 75–76
  recommendation for daily diet, 78
Dilation, 222, 225–26, 229–30
Disability benefits, 136–37
Discharge, See Early discharge.
Doctors
  family physician, 22
  pediatrician, 195–201
  preliminary consultations, 37–42
  role in prepping, 25–26
  team versus solo practice, 22–24
  See also Consultations.
Down's syndrome, 109–110
Dreams in pregnancy, 124–26
  research studies, 125–26
Drugs, 81–86
  aspirin, 84
  birth defects and, 81–82
  caffeine, 85–86
  over-the-counter drugs, 83–85
  vitamin/mineral supplements, 86
Due date, calculating, 56
Dystocia, 248

Early discharge, 18–20
  follow-up care and, 19
Eclampsia, 102
Effleurage, 206
Eisenstein, M., 51–52
Electronic Fetal Monitoring (EFM), 30–33
  effect on woman in labor, 32–33
  external monitor, 31
  internal monitor, 31
  purpose of, 30
Emotions
  postpartum depression, 264–66
  postpartum period, 261–63
  See also Pregnancy, emotional aspects.
Enema, rationale for, 27–28
Epidural, 217
Episiotomy
  anesthesia for, 218–19
  easing soreness of, 256
  necessity of, 242
Estriol testing, 112–13
Estrogen, 57
Exercise, 144–51
  benefits of, 145
  Kegel exercise, 150–51

Index

pelvic rock, 146–47
shoulder circling, 147
squatting, 148
tailor sitting, 149–50
External fetal monitor, 31

False labor, 220
Family-centered maternity
  care, 6–21
  birthing room, 8–11
  bonding time, 11–13
  early discharge, 18–20
  hospital programs for, 25
  Leboyer method, 20–21
  rooming-in, 14–16
  sibling participation
    visitation, 16–18
Family practice, 22
Fathers
  bottlefeeding and, 194
  breastfeeding and, 191
  Caesarean birth and, 251–52
  couvade syndrome, 118
  emotions and pregnancy,
    118, 121–24
  husband-coached childbirth,
    207
  participation of, 6–7
Fatigue, 59, 66–67
Feeding, newborns, 275
Fencing reflex, 274
Fetal Alcohol Syndrome
  (FAS), 89–90
Fetal development
  first trimester, 56, 58
  second trimester, 58, 60
  third trimester, 60, 62
Fetopelvic disproportion, 248
Fetoscope, 31
Fever, 99
Folic acid, 79–80
Front carriers, choosing, 172
Fruits/vegetables, 77
Furniture/equipment, 162–87
  baby seat, 177–78
  bath, 167–68
  car seat, 168–70
  carriages, 172–74
  crib/cradle/bassinet, 162–65
  drug store items, 186–87
  front/back carriers, 170–72
  high chair, 180–81
  layette, 182–86
  play yard, 178–80
  strollers, 174–77

Genetic testing, *See*
  Amniocentesis.
Gentle Birth Book, The
  (Berezin), 21
Gestational diabetes, 93
Gillman, R., 125
Glands of Montgomery, 59
Golf, 155
Gonorrhea, detection during
  pregnancy, 95
Gowns, choosing, 183–84
Grains, 77
Group practice, advantages/
  disadvantages of, 23

HCG, 59
  nausea and, 64
Headache, 99
Health insurance, 137

Heart rate
　auscultation, 31–32
　Electronic Fetal Monitoring, 30–33
Heartburn, 63, 68–69
Hemorrhoids, 63, 71–72
Herpes, venereal, 95
High chair, choosing, 180–81
Hillard, P., 26
Home birth, 50–53
　opponents/proponents of, 51–52
　screening for, 52
Hormonal changes, in pregnancy, 57, 59
Hospitals, 24–25
　family-centered options, 25
　midwifery programs, 43
　small hospitals, 24
　teaching hospitals, 24

Induced labor, 250–51
Insomnia, 67
Internal fetal monitor, 31
International Childbirth Education Association, 35
Intravenous, 28–30
　woman's mobility and, 30
Involution, 258
Iron, 78–79

Jogging, 154

Karmel, M., 206
Kegel exercise, 150–51, 256
Kennell, J., 11

Kimonos/saques, choosing, 184
Kitzinger, S., 209
Klaus, M., 11

Labor, 219–47
　active phase, 229–36
　arriving at birth setting, 233
　calling the caregiver, 231
　delivery of placenta, 244–45
　dreams in pregnancy and, 126
　dystocia, 248
　eating/drinking and, 29
　episiotomy, 241
　first stage of, 226–37
　induced, 250–51
　latent phase, 226–29
　onset of, 222–25
　positions in, 239–41
　prelabor, 220–21
　purpose of, 222
　pushing during, 238–40
　recovery period, 245–46
　rupturing of membranes, 222–25
　second stage of, 238–44
　shaking after delivery, 245
　squatting, 239–40
　third stage of, 244–47
　transition phase, 236–37
　See also Obstetrical procedures; Premature labor.
La Leche League, 190–92
Lamaze, F., 205–206, 208
Lap pads, 185

Index

Latent phase of labor, 226–29
Layette, essential items, 182–86
Leboyer birth, 20–21
Leg cramps, 69–70
Liquids, 77–78
Lithotomy position, 239–41
Lochia, 259

Maternity leave, 138
Medication, 213–19
  analgesia, 215–16
  anesthesia, 216–19
  Demerol, 215
  intravenous and, 29
Membranes, rupturing of, 222–25
Milk/dairy products, 76–77
Mood swings, 117–18
Moro reflex, 273
Movement of fetus, 61
Mucous plug, loss of, 221

Narcan, 216
Natural Childbirth (Dick-Read), 205
Natural childbirth, 203
  meaning of, 204
  See also Prepared childbirth.
Nausea, 57, 59, 64–66
  relief of, 65–66
Nesting interest, 221
Newborn, 269–77
  appearance of, 269–71
  bathing, 276–77
  behavior after birth, 12
  feeding, 275
  reflexes, 272–74
  senses, 271–72
  sleeping, 274–75
Nonroutine tests, 107–114
  alpha-fetoprotein (AFP) testing, 112
  amniocentesis, 109–111
  estriol testing, 112–13
  nonstress test, 113
  stress test, 113–14
  ultrasound, 108–109
Nonstress test, 113
Nurse-midwife, 42–46
  history of, 44–45
  philosophy of, 42
  physician back-up, 43–44
  source for finding of, 46
Nutritional supplements, 78–80
  folic acid, 79–80
  iron, 78–79
  multivitamin-mineral supplements, 80

Obesity, pregnancy and, 74–75
Obstetrical procedures, 25–33
  Electronic Fetal Monitoring (EFM), 30–33
  enema, 27–28
  intravenous, 28–30
  physician's role in, 26
  prepping, 25–26
  pubic shave, 27
Organizations as referral sources, 35–36
Oxytocin, 258
  stress test, 113–14

Pap smear, 95–96
Paracervical block, 218
Parent support groups as referral sources, 36
Pediatrician, 195–201
  considerations in choice of, 197–201
Perineal block, 218
Physician/hospital care, 21–33
  family physician, 22
  hospital, 24–25
  obstetrical procedures, 25–33
  preliminary consultations, 37–42
  team versus solo practice, 22–24
Pitocin, 250
Placenta, delivery of, 244–45
Placenta previa, 103–104
  abruptio placenta, 103–104
  cigarette smoking and, 88
Play yard, choosing, 178–180
Postmature syndrome, 107
  estriol testing, 112–13
Postpartum depression, 264–66
  mother-child separation and, 14–15
Postpartum period, 254–69
  body in, 258–59
  checkup, 259–60
  depression, 264–66
  emotional aspects, 261–63
  lochia (postpartum bleeding), 259
  post-delivery discomforts, 256–57
  sex, 267–69
Preeclampsia, 102
Pregnancy Discrimination Act, 136, 138–39
Pregnancy, emotional aspects, 115–34
  dreams, 124–26
  emotional changeability, 115–16
  first trimester and, 117–18
  second trimester and, 119–22
  sex, 127–34
  third trimester and, 112–24
Pregnancy, physical aspects, 54–114
  alcohol use, 89–90
  backache, 69
  cigarette smoking, 86–89
  complications, 100–107
  constipation, 67–68
  diet, 75–78
  drugs, 81–86
  due date calculation, 56
  exercise, 144–51
  fatigue, 66–67
  fetal development, 56, 58, 60, 62
  first trimester, 57, 59
  heartburn, 68–69
  hemorrhoids, 71–72
  insomnia, 67
  leg cramps, 69–70
  nausea, 64–66
  nonroutine tests, 107–114
  nutritional supplements, 78–80

Index

prenatal care, 90–98
second trimester, 61, 63
sports, 151–55
travel, 155–60
varicose veins, 70–71
warning signs, 98–99
weight gain, 72–75
work and, 135–44
Premature labor, 105–107
inhibition of, 106
Premature rupture of the membranes (PROM), 104–105
Prenatal care, 90–98
first visit, 91–92
routine tests, 92–96
visits for, 96–98
Prepared childbirth, 203–213
classes for, 210–12
Fernand Lamaze, 205–206, 208
Grantley Dick-Read, 204–205
meaning of, 203
Robert Bradley, 206–209
Sheila Kitzinger, 209
Preparing for baby, 161–201
bottle/breast combination, 194–205
bottlefeeding, 192–94
breastfeeding, 187–92
furniture/equipment, 162–87
Prepping, 25–26
See also Obstetrical procedures.
Progesterone, 57
Protein foods, 75–76

Psychosexual approach to birth, 209
Pubic shave, rationale for, 27
Pudendal block, 218
Pushing during labor, 238–40

Recovery period, 245–46
Referral sources, 33–36
friends/relatives, 34–35
organizations, 35–36
Reflexes of newborn, 272–74
crying, 273
grasping, 273
Moro (startle) reflex, 273
rooting, 272
sneezing/coughing/yawning, 272–73
stepping/crawling, 273
tonic neck (fencing) reflex, 274
Rh disease, 100–101
amniocentesis and, 111
RhoGAM, 100–101
Rh factor, test for, 93
Ritodrine, for premature labor, 106
Rooming-in, 14–16
breastfeeding and, 15
Rooting reflex, 272
Routine tests, 92–96
blood count, 93–94
blood type/Rh factor, 93
pap smear, 95–96
rubella, 94
for sexually transmitted diseases, 94–95
urinalysis, 92–93
Rubella, test for, 94

Senses of newborn, 271–72
"Sensitive period" after birth, 11–12
Sex, 127–34
  abstinence from, 127–28
  air embolism danger, 130
  in first trimester, 128–30
  in last weeks of pregnancy, 133
  in postpartum period, 267–69
  in second trimester, 130–31
  in third trimester, 131–34
Sexually transmitted diseases, tests for, 94–95
Shaking after delivery, 245
Sibling participation/visitation, 16–18
  advantages of, 17–18
  preparation for, 17
  types of, 18
Sleeping, newborns, 274–75
Speech, blurred, 99
Spina bifida, test for, 112
Spinal, 217–18
Sports, 151–55
  bicycle riding, 153
  bowling, 154
  golf, 155
  jogging, 154
  swimming, 152–53
  tennis, 153–54
Squatting, 239–40
Stress test, 113–14
Stretchies, choosing, 183
Stroller, choosing, 174–77
Sweaters, choosing, 184
Swimming, 152–53

Syphilis, detection during pregnancy, 94–95

Teaching hospitals, 24
Tennis, 153–54
Teratogens, 82
Tests, *See* Nonroutine tests; Routine tests.
Thalidomide, 81
Thank You, Dr. Lamaze (Karmel), 206
Tonic neck reflex, 274
Touch relaxation, 209
Towels/washcloths, 185–86
Toxemia, 75, 102–103
  eclampsia, 102
  preeclampsia, 102
  signs of, 93
Transducer, fetal monitor and, 31
Transition phase of labor, 236–37
Travel, 155–60
  best time for, 155–56
  modes of transportation, 157–59
  tips for, 159–60

Ultrasound, 108–109
Undershirts, choosing, 182
Urinalysis, 92–93
Urination, frequent, 57, 61, 67
  post-delivery, 256–57
Uterus, post-delivery, 258

Vaginal bleeding, 98–99
Vaginal discharge, 99

Index

Varicose veins, 63, 70–71
Vision, blurred, 99
Vitamin/mineral supplements,
   excessive doses, 86
Vitamins, *See* Nutritional
   supplements.
Vomiting, 99

Warning signs during
   pregnancy, 98–99
Weight gain, 72–75
  overweight and, 74
  recommendations, 73–74
  toxemia and, 75, 102
  See also Diet.
Work, 135–44
  benefits, 136–37
  co-workers, 143–44
  legal rights, 136
  maternity leave, 138
  modifications in routine
    during pregnancy, 142–43
  occupational safety, 138–39
  telling the boss, 140–42

About the Author

Leah Kalnitz Yarrow was an associate editor of *Parents* Magazine for more than four years. She is now a freelance writer. Married and the mother of two, Leah makes her home in Chicago.

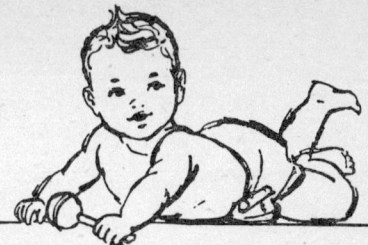

BRINGING UP BABY

A series of practical baby care and family living guides developed with the staff of *Parents Magazine*. Explains both the *whys* and *how-to's* of infant care.

Available at your bookstore or use this coupon.

___ ***PARENTS*™ BOOK FOR YOUR BABY'S FIRST YEAR**, Maja Bernath   30442   3.50
Recognizes the individuality of every child in his or her development and stresses flexibility in infant development. (July)

___ ***PARENTS*™ BOOK OF TOILET TEACHING**, Joanna Cole   30444   2.50
Tells you what to expect, with a step by step guide so that you and your child can relax — and get results. (August)

___ ***PARENTS*™ BOOK OF CHILDHOOD ALLERGIES**, Richard Graber   30443   2.95
With one in every six children suffering from one or more allergies, this book provides sound medical information, advice and emotional support. (September)

___ ***PARENTS*™ BOOK OF BREAST FEEDING**, Susan Trien   30445   2.95
A step by step guide beginning with the decision to nurse all the way to the weaning process. (October)

BB   BALLANTINE MAIL SALES
Dept. TA, 201 E. 50th St., New York, N.Y. 10022

Please send me the BALLANTINE or DEL REY BOOKS I have checked above. I am enclosing $_____ (add 50¢ per copy to cover postage and handling). Send check or money order — no cash or C.O.D.'s please. Prices and numbers are subject to change without notice.

Name_____

Address_____

City_____ State_____ Zip Code_____

Allow at least 4 weeks for delivery.

TA-66